MIX
Papier aus verantwortungsvollen Quellen
Paper from responsible sources
FSC® C105338

Dr. Kuldeep Dhama
Dr. Basavaraj Patthi
Dr. Ashish Singla

Topical Fluorides

A literature review

Anchor Academic Publishing

Dhama, Kuldeep, Patthi, Basavaraj, Singla, Ashish: Topical Fluorides. A literature review, Hamburg, Anchor Academic Publishing 2017

Buch-ISBN: 978-3-96067-142-8
PDF-eBook-ISBN: 978-3-96067-642-3
Druck/Herstellung: Anchor Academic Publishing, Hamburg, 2017

Bibliografische Information der Deutschen Nationalbibliothek:
Die Deutsche Nationalbibliothek verzeichnet diese Publikation in der Deutschen Nationalbibliografie; detaillierte bibliografische Daten sind im Internet über http://dnb.d-nb.de abrufbar.

Bibliographical Information of the German National Library:
The German National Library lists this publication in the German National Bibliography. Detailed bibliographic data can be found at: http://dnb.d-nb.de

All rights reserved. This publication may not be reproduced, stored in a retrieval system or transmitted, in any form or by any means, electronic, mechanical, photocopying, recording or otherwise, without the prior permission of the publishers.

Das Werk einschließlich aller seiner Teile ist urheberrechtlich geschützt. Jede Verwertung außerhalb der Grenzen des Urheberrechtsgesetzes ist ohne Zustimmung des Verlages unzulässig und strafbar. Dies gilt insbesondere für Vervielfältigungen, Übersetzungen, Mikroverfilmungen und die Einspeicherung und Bearbeitung in elektronischen Systemen.

Die Wiedergabe von Gebrauchsnamen, Handelsnamen, Warenbezeichnungen usw. in diesem Werk berechtigt auch ohne besondere Kennzeichnung nicht zu der Annahme, dass solche Namen im Sinne der Warenzeichen- und Markenschutz-Gesetzgebung als frei zu betrachten wären und daher von jedermann benutzt werden dürften.

Die Informationen in diesem Werk wurden mit Sorgfalt erarbeitet. Dennoch können Fehler nicht vollständig ausgeschlossen werden und die Diplomica Verlag GmbH, die Autoren oder Übersetzer übernehmen keine juristische Verantwortung oder irgendeine Haftung für evtl. verbliebene fehlerhafte Angaben und deren Folgen.

Alle Rechte vorbehalten

© Anchor Academic Publishing, Imprint der Diplomica Verlag GmbH
Hermannstal 119k, 22119 Hamburg
http://www.diplomica-verlag.de, Hamburg 2017
Printed in Germany

ACKNOWLEDGMENTS

"What is a teacher? I'll tell you: it isn't someone who teaches something, but someone who inspires the student to give of her best in order to discover what she already knows."

Paulo Coelho, The Witch of Portobello

There is not a more pleasing exercise of the mind than gratitude which is accompanied with such an inward satisfaction that the duty is sufficiently rewarded by the performance. This dissertation would not have been composed and completed without the efforts of many people, to whom I offer my most sincere and heartfelt thanks. Successful completion of a chore is often due to the fact that the individual has been blessed by the Almighty and fortunate to be amidst the individuals with whom he has been associated. I would never have been able to finish my dissertation without the guidance of my Guide and my Lecturers, support from my family and help from friends.

Nevertheless, failure in my ability to express what I feel cannot refrain me from saluting and thanking me to dedicate this dissertation to the invaluable guidance and support rendered to me by my esteemed mentor and Guide, **Dr. Basavaraj Patthi** (Prof. & Head of the Dept.) Dept. of Public Health Dentistry, D.J College of Dental Sciences and Research, Modinagar who motivates and encourages the ability in oneself to create the best of one's future. **"Sir, I am especially grateful to you for your devotion to your students' knowledge and growth. Your emphasis on punctuality, perseverance and being systematic has helped me in improving myself continuously. I am blessed to have you as my mentor who bind us together like a family and has been there for us in our thick and thin. You have always strived to bring out the best of me both as a student and as a person. Sir, your pearls of wisdom coupled with valuable criticism have contributed largely in my way to completion of this work. Without your immense knowledge, inspirational thoughts and indispensable support my dissertation could never have been possible. Thank You for understanding my apprehensions and raising my morale by showing me the right direction always."**

It is with deep humbleness, privilege and honor to pay regards, supreme sincerity and heartfelt appreciation to my Co-Guide, **Dr. Ashish Singla** (Reader, Dept. of Public Health

Dentistry) whose dedication and perfectionism towards work has always been an inspiration to me and encourages me to be more responsible and efficient towards my work. **"Thank you Ashish sir for your valuable suggestions, incessant cooperation, continuous support and inexhaustible guidance and for helping me at each and every step of my work by checking minutest details with your endless patience and knowledge. which made my dissertation to see the light of the day."**

With deep gratitude and regards I wish to express my indebtedness to my revered teacher **Dr. Ritu Gupta** (Senior Lecturers, Dept. of Public Health Dentistry) for their constant enthusiasm and valuable suggestions. **"Thank you ma'am for clearing my unending doubts with your intelligence and helping me to improve my work . Thank you ma'am for your comprehensive outlook, tireless efforts and relentless help and keeping the patience from inception to completion of this dissertation."**

I would also like to thank **Dr. Malik Arjun** (Senior Lecturer) and Dr. Sunil (BDS lecturer) for their constant help and support. **"Thank you sir for your constant support."**

With most sincerity I would like to pay my profound gratitude to the **Dean** and **Pricipal**, **Dr. Reena R Kumar**, who has been a fountain head of knowledge, a symbol of zest and an inspiration to millions. **"Thank you ma'am for having the integrity, strength and courage to lead me down the right path and showing me how I can be confident in my abilities."**

I would also like to express my heartfelt gratitude to **Dr. Smriti Jassar**, **CEO** for their support and help.

My sincere thanks to Administrator **Dr. Navneet sharma** for his support. My heartfelt gratitude to all the administrative staff for helping me in this journey.

A big thanks to my Co P.G.s **Dr. Lav Kumar Niraj** and **Dr.Irfan Ali** for being the most awesome, coolest and loving batchmates one can be blessed with." Thank you for being there for me whenever I needed."

I also like to express my heartfelt thanks and regard to my seniors **Dr. Monika prasad** and **Dr. Jishnu krishna kumar** for being the most helpful and supportive seniors. You have been the best of mentors to me and have guided me with your at every stage of my P.G life both personally and professionally with your immense knowledge along with parental affection full of constant encouragement.

I thank all my wonderful and loving juniors **Dr. Devanshu**, **Dr. Mohnish** and **Dr. Yashasvini** for their valuable help, assistance and co-operation. They altogether contribute to the memories which I will cherish for lifetime. **"Thank you Devanshu and Mohnish, for being the most sincere junior and helping me with endless patience and smile".**

A heartfelt gratitude to all the B.D.S students for their help. A sincere thanks to the attendants **Anu** and **Kallu** for their help and support.

I am greatly indebted to my **Father, Mr. Jitender Singh** and my **Mother, Mrs. Bimlesh** who made it possible for me to live my dream.

I express my thanks and regards to my Brother in law and Sister **Mr. Munesh Panwar** and **Mrs. Neetu Panwar** for their unconditional love and all time blessings. **"Thank you Jiju and Dii for being my friends, philosopher and guide and showering all your love on me and making me feel special."**

Friends are the family we choose for ourselves. A good friendship is indeed something to savor and protect and without their support this dissertation would not have been possible. I express my thanks and love to my best friends **Dr. Ankan Chaudhary** and **Nirdosh Singh** for being the most co-operative and lovely member of my life. **"Thank you for all your love and concern towards me. You have done all the possibilities to bring a smile on my face even in the hardest of times."**

I also thank my batchmates **Dr. Rohan Chaudhary** and **Dr. Nitin Som** who being my best friends have been a great support in all my struggles. **"Thank you guys for boosting my confidence in the times whenever I felt blue and for being the part of all the best moments of my P.G life."**

Also, I am thankful to **M/S Jain computer works**, Modinagar, for patiently helping in the final formatting of my dissertation

With folded hands I bow to **THE ALMIGHTY** who has been giving me everything to accomplish this thesis: Patience, health, wisdom, and blessing. I also thank him for making all the above mentioned names my part of life and giving me the opportunity to undertake this work and complete it successfully.

Kuldeep Dhama

TABLE OF CONTENTS

1. INTRODUCTION 7
2. DEFINITIONS 11
3. CLASSIFICATION 15
4. MODE OF ACTION OF TOPICAL FLUORIDES 16
5. HISTORY OF FLUORIDE 17
6. MILESTONE STUDIES 25
7. HOME APPLIED / SELF APPLIED 27
8. PROFESSIONALLY APPLIED 42
9. METHODS OF APPLICATION OF TOPICAL FLUORIDE 59
10. RECOMMENDATION IN USE OF PROFESSIONALLY APPLIED TOPICAL FLUORIDES 62
11. RECENT ADVANCE IN TOPICAL FLUORIDES 66
12. DISCUSSION 68
13. CONCLUSIONS 72
14. BIBLIOGRAPHY 75

INTRODUCTION

Dental caries is a multi factorial, bacterial, chronic infection that affects millions of people in the world and has become a public health problem. Also referred to as tooth decay, this disease is one of the most common disorders throughout the world, second only to the common cold. Dental caries is the most common chronic childhood disease in the United States and is 5 to 7 times more common than asthma. According to the World Oral Health Report in 2003, dental caries affect 60-80% of school children and a vast majority of adults. Dental caries is a chronic bacterial infection of the hard tissue of the tooth that is characterized by alternating phases of demineralization and remineralization. Dental decay can lead to significant pain and dysfunction that can interfere with basic functions such as eating, sleeping, and speaking. If left untreated, dental caries can result in cavities forming and eventually tooth loss. Although the prevalence and severity of dental caries has decreased over the years, this disease can be better controlled with proper fluoride exposure[1].

With more than 50 years of clinical success, fluoride serves as the gold standard agent for preventing tooth decay[2]. Fluoride has both systemic and topical actions that are important in preventing dental caries. Systemically, fluoride acts on teeth before their eruption by being incorporated into the crystal structure of enamel and thus making this tissue more resistant to the caries process. In addition, fluoride limits the demineralization of enamel and promotes its remineralization into a stable crystal structure which is more caries resistant. Systemic fluoride therapy is most effective when it is initiated during the maturation of the primary and permanent teeth. The most common forms of systemic fluoride therapy include water fluoridation and dietary supplements[3]

Fluorides also act topically, (i.e., directly on erupted teeth), by promoting remineralization and, to a lesser degree, through antibacterial action. These topical effects are significant and exposure of the tooth surface to low, regular doses of fluoride may be as critical in preventing caries as is fluoride ingested during tooth formation[2,3]. Topical fluorides generally fall into two categories: (a) self applied – e.g. toothpaste and mouthrinse, and (b) professionally applied – e.g. solutions, gels, foams and varnish. Professionally applied fluoride varnish, gel and foam are high concentration fluoride vehicles which are applied by healthcare professionals intermittently for caries prevention. Their caries preventive effect is topical and although they should not be ingested, small amounts will inevitably be swallowed by patients[4].

The fluoride solutions which are commonly used includes 2% Sodium Fluoride and 8% Stannous Fluoride solution. Chronologically, neutral 2 percent sodium fluoride solution (9040 ppm Fluoride ion) applied by the "paint-on" technique was the first topical Fuoride to be used in public health programs. Both sodium fluoride and stannous fluoride in solutions of various concentrations have been used as topical agents, and their effectiveness as dental caries preventives among school children has been reported. A series of four applications of 2 percent solution of sodium fluoride to the teeth of children has been shown to reduce the incidence of dental caries by approximately 40 percent[5]

a) Knutson, J. W., and Armstrong, W. D.: The effect of topically applied sodium fluoride on dental caries experience. I. Report of findings for the first study year. Pub. Health Rep. 58: 17011715, Nov. 19,1943. (2)

b) Galagan, D. J., and Knutson, J. W.: The effect of topically applied fluorides on dental caries experience. V. Report of findings with two, four and six applications of sodium fluoride and of lead fluoride. Pub. Health Rep. 62: 1477-1483, Oct. 10, 1947).

Reports on the effectiveness of 2 and 8 percent concentrations of stannous fluoride solution, topically applied, have varied widely among different workers

a) Howell, C. L., Gish, C. W., Smiley, R. D., and Muhler, J. C.: Effect of topically applied stannous fluoride on dental caries experience in children. J. Am. Dent. A. 50: 14-17, January 1955. (4)

b) Gish, C. W., Howell, C. L., and Muhler, J. C.: Effect of a single topical application of stannous fluoride on caries experience. International Association of Dental Research, 34th Meeting, March 1956. (Abstract.) (5)

c) Gish, C. W., Howell, C. L., and Muhler, J. C.: A new approach to the topical application of fluorides for the reduction of dental caries in children. J. Dent Res. 36: 784-786, October 1957

The concentration of fluoride in gel typically ranges from 5,000 ppm to 12,300 ppm. It has a viscous texture which allows its professional application in a tray, with cotton wool or with dental floss. The most commonly used formulation of gel is 1.23% acidulated phosphate fluoride (APF) containing 12,300 ppm fluoride. A typical fluoride gel treatment using APF gel involves the application of 3 to 5 ml of gel, containing 36.9 to 61.5mg of fluoride ion. It has been reported that 2.8% to 78% of the initial dose of fluoride may be retained following fluoride gel application. The amount of fluoride retained depends on the amount of gel used, the age of the subject and the application technique[6].

Fluoride varnishes may be aqueous solutions (e.g. Bifluorid) or non-aqueous solutions of natural resins (e.g. Duraphat, Lawefluor). Resin-based varnishes have a sticky texture, which prolongs the contact time between the fluoride and the enamel. The concentration of fluoride in varnish ranges from 1,000 ppm (Fluor Protector) to 56,300 ppm (Bifluorid 12). The fluoride formulations that are found in most commercially available varnishes are:

a) 5% sodium fluoride (Duraphat, Colgate Palmolive)

b) 1% difluorsilane (Fluor Protector, Ivoclar-Vivadent)

c) 6% sodium fluoride plus 6% calcium fluoride (Biflucrid 12, VOCO GmbH)

Although the fluoride concentration of varnishes is typically very high, the nature of varnish lends itself to controlled, precise application to specific tooth surfaces. A single 0.25 ml application of fluoride varnish with 22,600 ppm F contains 5.65 mg of fluoride ion, which is well below the probably toxic dose (PTD) for fluoride of 5 mg/kg body weight72, even if all the varnish dispensed is swallowed[5]

Fluoride foam is a relatively recent product which has the same fluoride concentration (12,300 ppm), pH (3–4) and method of application (tray) as conventional APF gel. The advantage of foam over gel is that less material needs to be used, and therefore the patient's risk of ingesting excess fluoride is reduced[5,6].

Fluoride dentifrices have been shown in numerous clinical trials to be effective anticaries agents and have been recognized as a major cause of the remarkable decline in caries prevalence in many developed countries . Dentifrices have been widely adopted around the world as the principle means of delivering topical fluoride and obtaining caries preventive benefits. Over 95% of all dentifrices,Studies showed that daily toothbrushing using fluoridated toothpaste (1000 ppm F) could arrest non-cavitated lesions as well as dentin caries lesions . Toothpaste containing higher fluoride concentration, e.g. 5000 ppm, has better results in remineralizing carious lesions compared to those containing 1000 ppm . F Recently it has been demonstrated that elevated fluoride products like dentifrices with 5000 ppm NaF or amine fluoride or oral hygiene tablets directly dissolved in saliva with 4350ppm NaF enhance remineralization of advanced enamel lesions and result in increased bioavailability of fluoride in saliva [5].

Although there is documented literature on the use of topical fluorides, the issues needs to be futher researched based on the recent documented literature and guidelines regarding use of topical fluorides hence the present review was conducted with the aim to review the available literature on the use and effectiveness of different topical fluorides used in dentistry

DEFINITIONS

Fluoride [floor´īd]: Any binary compound of fluorine.

fluoride poisoning: A toxic condition that sometimes occurs with ingestion of excessive fluoride.

Acute fluoridepoisoning: Involves an immediate physiological reaction, with nausea, vomiting, hypersalivation, abdominal pain, anddiarrhea.

Chronic fluoride poisoning: Is a physiological reaction to long term exposure to high levels of fluoride and is characterized by dental FLUOROSIS, skeletal FLUOROSIS, and kidney damage. Called also fluorosis.

Systemic fluoride : A fluoride ingested in water, supplements, or some other form.

Topical fluoride: A fluoride applied directly to the teeth, especially of children, in a DENTAL CARIES prevention program.

BY: Miller-Keane Encyclopedia and Dictionary of Medicine, Nursing, and Allied Health, Seventh Edition. © 2003 by Saunders, an imprint of Elsevier, Inc. All rights reserved.

Fluoride:

1. A compound of fluorine with a metal, a nonmetal, or an organic radical.

2. The anion of fluorine; inhibits enolase; found in bone and tooth apatite; fluoride has a cariostatic effect; high levelsare toxic.

BY: Farlex Partner Medical Dictionary © Farlex 2012

Fluoride:

An anion of fluorine. Fluoride compounds are introduced into drinking water or applied directly to the teeth to prevent toothdecay.

BY: Mosby's Medical Dictionary, 9th edition. © 2009, Elsevier.

Fluoride:

A compound of fluorine with a metal, a nonmetal, or an organic radical; the anion of fluorine; inhibits enolase; found inbone and tooth apatite; fluoride has a cariostatic effect; high levels are toxic.

BY: Medical Dictionary for the Health Professions and Nursing © Farlex 2012

Fluoride:

A compound of fluorine that replaces hydroxyl groups in teeth and bones and reduces the tendency to toothdecay. Its therapeutic use was discovered accidentally at Bauxite, Arkansas, when water containing fluoride was replacedby water lacking fluoride, resulting in an increase of dental cavities in children.

BY: Collins Dictionary of Biology, 3rd ed. © W. G. Hale, V. A. Saunders, J. P. Margham 2005

Fluoride:

A chemical compound containing fluorine that is used to treat water or applied directly to teeth to prevent decay.

BY: Gale Encyclopedia of Medicine. Copyright 2008 The Gale Group, Inc. All rights reserved.

Fluoride:

A mineral important in bone formation used for the treatment of osteoporosis and prevention of tooth decay.Overdose can produce tooth mottling, joint pain, stomach pain, and nausea.

BY: Jonas: Mosby's Dictionary of Complementary and Alternative Medicine. (c) 2005, Elsevier.

Fluoride(s):

A salt of hydrofluoric acid, commonly sodium or stannous (tin).

Fluoride dietary supplements:

The orally administered nutritional additives of the chemical fluoride; often taken by individuals without regular access to a fluoridated water supply; available as chewable tablets, drops, pills, and in combination with vitamin supplements. See also fluoride drops.

Fluoride drops:

A supplemental liquid form of the chemical fluoride. They can be administered to children from 6 months to 3 years of age but are not usually recommended because most children are exposed to normal levels of fluoride in their water systems at home and school and in their beverages.

Fluoride, stannous:

A compound of tin and fluorine used in dentifrices to prevent caries.

Fluoride tablets/lozenges:

The supplemental forms of the chemical fluoride. Tablets must be chewed, and lozenges must be held in the oral cavity until dissolved in order to benefit from the fluoride's contact with the teeth.

Fluoride toxicity:

Poisoning as a result of ingesting too much fluoride. Symptoms range from upset stomach to death.

Fluoride varnish:

A topical resin containing fluoride that is thinly applied to the tooth surface and used as a preventive treatment for caries. Can also be used as a desensitizing agent to treat dentinal

Fluorides, topical:

The salts of hydrofluoric acid (usually sodium or tin salts) that may be applied in solution to the exposed dental surfaces to prevent dental caries and promote remineralization. They can be applied by trays or mouthrinses or by techniques such as paint-on.

Fluorides, topical, paint-on technique:

A professionally administered procedure in which the exposed dental surfaces are coated with a fluoride solutionor gel or varnish to prevent caries and promote remineralization.

BY: Mosby's Dental Dictionary, 2nd edition. © 2008 Elsevier, Inc. All rights reserved.

Fluoride: Any binary compound of fluorine.

BY: Saunders Comprehensive Veterinary Dictionary, 3 ed. © 2007 Elsevier, Inc. All rights reserved

CLASSIFICATION

TOPICAL FLUORIDES

1. HOME USE (SELF APPLICATION)

- FLUORIDE DENTRIFICES
- FLUORIDE MOUTHRINSES
- FLUORIDE GELS
- FLUORIDE FOAM

2. PROFESSIONALLY APPLIED

- FLUORIDE GEL AND SOLUTION
  - SODIUM FLUORIDE (NaF)
  - STANNOUS FLUORIDE (SnF2)
  - ACIDULATED PHOSPHATE FLUORIDE (APF)
- FLUORIDE VARNISH
- FLUORIDE FORM
- FLUORIDE PROPHYLACTIC PASTE

MODE OF ACTION OF TOPICAL FLUORIDES

The primary and most important action of fluoride is topical, when the fluoride ion is present in the saliva in the appropriate concentration[7]. Hydroxyapatite is the main mineral responsible for building the permanent tooth enamel after the development of the teeth is finished[8]. During tooth growth, the enamel is constantly exposed to numerous demineralization processes, but also important remineralization processes, if the appropriate ions are present in the saliva. These processes can either weaken or strengthen the enamel. The presence of fluoride in an acidic environment reduces the dissolution of calcium hydroxyapatite .The main action is inhibition of demineralization of enamel, which is carried out through different mechanisms. There are different cariogenic bacteria in the plaque fluid the most important being S. mutans. When bacteria metabolize sugars, they produce lactic acid which decreases the pH in saliva. When the pH falls below the critical level of hydroxyapatite (pH 5.5), the process of demineralization of enamel takes place and caries is formed. At the beginning, the process is reversible and it is possible to reduce the formation of new lesions with appropriate preventive measures. If fluoride is present in plaque fluid, it will reduce the demineralization, as it will adsorb into the crystal surface and protect crystals from dissolution. Because the fluoride ion coating is only partial, the uncoated parts of the crystal will undergo dissolution on certain parts of the tooth, if the pH falls below level 5.5. When the pH rises above the critical level of 5.5, the increased level of fluoride ion leads to remineralization, because it absorbs itself into the enamel and forms fluorhydroxyapatite[7,8]. After repeated cycles of demineralization and remineralization, the outer parts of enamel may change and become more resistant to the acidic environment due to a lowered critical pH level of newly formed crystals (pH 4.5) . The most important effect of fluoride on caries progression is thus on demineralization and remineralization processes. It has also been proposed, that the fluoride ion can affect the physiology of microbial cells, which can indirectly affect demineralization. Fluoride ions affect bacterial cells through several mechanisms. One of them being a direct inhibition of cellular enzymes – glycolytic enzymes, H+ATPases). It affects cellular membrane permeability and also lowers cytoplasmic pH, resulting in a decrease in acid production from glycolysis[7].

Fluoride prevents caries mainly by its topical effect . Dental caries result when plaque, a sticky film of bacteria on the surface of the tooth, feeds on sugar and food residue to produce acid, which dissolves the surface of the tooth(demineralization). Bathing the surface of the tooth with as little as 1 ppm of fluoride causes a dramatic decrease in enamel solubility. Ingested fluoride, on the other hand, has little effect on caries, but contributes significantly to the development of fluorosis[9].

HISTORY OF FLUORIDE. [10,11]

Figure 1: History of Fluoride[10,11]

1530	Fluorine in the form of fluorspar was first described by a German physician George Bauer, through his book "De re metallica".
1803	Count Carlo Morozzo of Italy found elephant fossil skeleton, which contained organic substance, carbonic acid, fluoric acid.
1805	Morichini found fluoric acid in human teeth and claimed that fluoric acid is a main component of dental enamel.
1805	Joseph Louis Gay-Lussac claimed that the enamel of teeth is especially rich in "fluate" of lime as the fluoride was called then and the canine teeth contain more of the fluate than the other teeth.
1806	Neither tooth enamel nor bones revealed the slightest traces of fluoric acid after ashing.
1807	Detection of fluoride in samples of bones and teeth by Jöns Jacob Berzelius.
1820	Diluted fluoric acid might dissolve in the digestive tract any accidentally swallowed pieces of glass as found by W. Krimer.
1822	Berzelius discovered fluoride 3.3 mg/l in the water of Carlsbad.
1827	Fluoride was detected by the etching-of-glass test. Gustav Rose gave the formula of apatite ($CaF^4 + 3\ Ca^3P^2$)
1833	Berzelius stated that bones and teeth contain up to a few tenths of a percent fluoride.
1839	The chemist Friedrich Wöhler proposed a new method for fluoride estimation: silica is added to every sample along with sulfuric acid.
1840	Morichini and Gay-Lussac (1805) - calcium fluoride seems to be able to substitute for calcium phosphate in the bones and teeth.
1842	Girardin and Preisser were unable to find the slightest trace of fluoric acid in human and animal bones.
1844	Antoine Malagou the French dentist recommended use of fluorides for the preparation of dental fillings.

1849	W. Heintz carried out the etching-of-glass test, with powdered bone -proof of the presence of fluoride.
1851	George Wilson found fluoride in several waters, in sea-water, in plants, urine, blood and milk.
1852	Wilson presented new methods for the detection of fluoride in the presence of silica which usually makes recognition of fluoride very difficult
1853	Fluorine was found in fossil bones of Nebraska.
1854	Fremy claimed that recent bones contain very low and variable amounts of fluoride. Fossil bones contain more fluoride, silica in the form of quartz.
1856	Jerome Nicklès attributed to fluoride as "an importance it never had before in medicine and physiology" after its detection in various constituent of the body.
1857	Fluoride is present in glass in small amount or it's the constituent of etching chemical incoperated in to it
1862	Felix Hoppe could not detect any fluoride in the immature tooth enamel of newborn pigs but found in mature enamel of adult pigs, humans.
1866	Zalesky saw weight loss of glass plates due to formation of gaseous silicon fluoride developed from acid-treated samples.
1874	In January, 1874, Alvaro Francisco Carlos Reynosa, of France, did a Improvement in medical compounds on "Elixir" and "Sirup" containing fluoride of potassium, sodium or ammonium.
1875	According to Erhardt, that enamel is thinner if not enough fluoride is given but that the tooth may be kept healthy for a longer time if more fluoride is supplied.
1888	Albert Robin used to prescribe a fluoride (10 to 100 mgs. a day) to his patients as fluoride is to degrade the enzyme diastase against the unfavorable action of lactic and butyric ferments.
1889	Hugo Schulz demonstrated the toxicity of sodium fluoride in feeding experiments on several animal species.
1890	Fluorides and silicofluorides (in dilutions of 1: 1,000) were found to inhibit the development of certain infective germs in vitro and were useful as additives in the alcoholic fermentation process.

1891	J. Brandl & H. Tappeiner showed more fluoride in root than in crown and more in dentin than enamel.
1892	Crichton-Browne proved that the enamel of the teeth contains more fluorine, in the form of fluoride of calcium, than any other part of the body
1893	Wrampelmeyer analyzed the fluoride contents of sound versus diseased teeth of adults and children.
1894	Gabriel revealed that if there's any fluoride at all in bones and teeth, it is below 0.1%, and that, therefore, it is definitely of no importance
1897	A. Michel estimated the fluoride content of sound and carious teeth by Fresenius' method.
1899	Hempel and Scheffler modified Fresenius' method to separate carbon dioxide from the silicon fluoride in the course of the procedure.
1899	Heinrich Harms published his results obtained with a modification by Brandl of the Fresenius method to remove hydrochloric acid from the fumes
1903	After earlier reports that sodium fluoride inhibits bacterial metabolism, it came into use as a food preservative.
1904	Von Stubenrauch noticed anomalous development of teeth, faulty positions, heavy wear, and "a typical caries" in dog fed with lot of sodium fluoride.
1907	Albert Deninger, recommended calcium fluoride pills to prevent not only tooth decay but also appendicitis.
1908	Alphonse Brissemoret regarded calcium fluoride as as an important binding agent for the minerals of bones and teeth.
1909	Pharmaceutical Company of Berlin, patented a fluoride preparation from which the substance could be easily absorbed
1910	Another analysis of teeth performed by Gassmann using Walter Hempel's method revealed the same "fluoride" values in teeth as found earlier by other researchers using that procedure.

	Historic evolution of fluoride in dentistry
1901	Started with the arrival of Dr Fredrick Mckay in Colorado Springs, Colorado, USA, in 1901, He noticed stains on permanent teeth as "Colorado Stain". He called the stains later as "MOTTLED ENAMEL
1902	The first systemic endeavour to investigate this lesion was made by Colorado springs Dental Society in 1902
1908	Mckay presented a case at the annual meeting of State Dental Association in Boulder and he found that this condition was not only confined to Colorads, but extended to other towns as well
1912	Mckay came across the article written by Dr.J M Eager (1912) from Italy. Who reported that a high proportion of Italian residents in Nepal had ugly brown stain on their teeth known as Denti di chiaie.
1916	Mckay and Black examined 6,873 individual in USA and reported that an unknown causative factor of mottled enamel was possibly present in domestic water during the period of tooth calcification.
1930	Kemp and Mckay observed that no mottling occurred in people who grew up in Bauxite prior to 1909, the year in which Bauxite had changed its supply from shallow well to deep drilled wells
1931	Chirchill H V, after thorough spectragraphic analysis of the rare elements noted that fluoride was present in Bauxite water at a level of 13.7ppm
1931	"SHOE LATHER SURVEY" by Trendly H Dean.
1934	Trendly H Dean introduced mottling index which is popularly known as Dean's index for flourosis.
1942	The important milestone discovery was made by Dean et al that 1 ppm F In drinking water, 60% reduction in dental caries experience was observed
1945	World first artificial fluoridation plant at Grand rapids ,in January 25 was done in USA.
1946	Klein examined children of Japanese ancestry who had been transferred from a community containing 0.1 ppm flouride or less to Arizona, where the water contained 3 ppm of fluoride

1949	Russel examined caries in migrant children who lived in south Dakota with 1 ppm of fluoride in drinking water and had moved into the area containing only 0.2 ppm fluoride, resulted in progressive loss of cariostatic effect of fluoride
1969	Fluoridation was endorsed by the W H O and Dental prosthesis model base composition containing calcium fluoride, was made.
1971	Cements were produced by additions of stannous fluoride, stannous fluorozirconate, Indium fluorozirconate, Zirconium hexafluorogermanate, Indium hexafluorogermanate ort Zirconyl hexafluorogermanate.
1979	"Light curable acrylic dental composition with calcium fluoride pigment" was introduced.
1985	Fluoride interpolymeric resin was prepared
1987	Fluorine-containing dental materials", boron trifluoride which gives off fluoride upon contact with water.
1994	Process for preparing a ceramic material for use in dental fillings and dental crowns contains fluoroapatite.
1995	Fluoridation commemorative monument was dedicated in sept 1995 in Grandrapids, Michigan
1997	Introducing fluoride into glass, Aluminosilicate glass particles are fluoridated by stirring them into a solution of NH4-HF2, can be used in glass ionomer cement compositions with polyacrylic acid without tartaric acid or other chelating agent
2001	Fluoride-releasing amalgam dental restorative material.

Fluoride was first added to toothpaste in 1956 by Proctor and Gamble in the form of Crest toothpaste.

History of Fluoridation:

The study of fluoride in water began in the early 1900s with Dr. J.M. Eager, an American dentist of the Public Health Service stationed in Italy, and Dr. Fredrick McKay, a dentist in the United States. While Eager was stationed in Italy, he recorded dental-clinical reports of his examination of the deteriorated conditions of oral health among Italian emigrants. He found fine black horizontal lines on the teeth, which he described as a dental disease called "denti di Chiaie" (McClure, 1970). He noted the areas where he saw this unusual disease were near Naples, a region with volcanic formations. In 1901, he reported that local geological conditions had an impact on the Italian emigrants' teeth, as they drank water from nearby springs. At the same time, McKay noticed the same problem in the United States and devoted his time to resolving this disease. Though McKay was not aware of Eager's findings until ten years later, the report on Italian conditions was identical to what McKay saw in Colorado (Crain, Katz, & Rosenthal, 1969). McKay opened a dental office in Colorado in 1908 and noticed that many of his patients had brown, mottling stains on permanent teeth, which he called "Colorado Brown Stains" (McClure, 1970). As McKay looked into this matter, he first learned that the stain was widespread in many Rocky Mountain communities, but he could not find a cause (Crain, Katz, & Rosenthal, 1969). As McKay investigated these occurrences, he garnered the interest of Dr. Greene Vardiman Black, Dean of the Northwestern University Dental School in Chicago and a leading dental histologist. Working together in 1916, the two men described the mottle as a developmental disease that only affected the color of the teeth. They suspected that water was the cause, calling this the "waterborne hypothesis" (McClure, 1970). By this time, McKay had published his observation that mottled teeth also showed less tooth decay. However, he was so intent in finding the cause of the staining, he had ignored the significance of this discovery (Crain, Katz, & Rosenthal, 1969)[11].

In 1909, shallow wells in Bauxite, Arkansas were replaced with three deep wells, changing the water supply. Local dentist, Dr. F. L. Robertson noticed that children born after 1909 had stained teeth, whereas those born prior to 1909 did not (McClure, 1970). In 1926, Robertson asked the U.S. Public Health Service to investigate and in 1928 McKay and Dr. Grover A. Kempf started a survey. During this investigation, McKay traveled to Italy to observe the environs in which Eager had reported the same stains. He began his research around Naples and examined new cases of severe mottling on adult teeth in the city of Resina. McKay's research in Resina revealed that community members were drinking water piped from a mountain nearby, where previously they had been drinking water from a well. McKay conducted further research in rural districts and identified that people drinking out of private wells did not have the dental disease. Hence, his research provided some evidence for a waterborne contaminant forming within the earth and causing the staining (McClure, 1970). McKay had not yet determined what the stain-causing agent was. Because fluorine is a very active element, the ordinary chemical analysis that McKay performed was not able to isolate it (Crain, Katz, & Rosenthal, 1969).

While McKay failed to find the agent, Bauxite's water supply research caught the attention of H.V. Churchill, a chemist with the Aluminum Company of America (ALCOA). Churchill started researching the Bauxite water supply, believing there was a relationship between the staining on patients' teeth and aluminum. He ordered a sample of Bauxite's water from McKay and tested for rare elements that would go undetected in the usual chemical analysis (McNeil, 1985). The results spectrographically identified the presence of fluorine in Bauxite's water instead of aluminum (McClure, 1970). To confirm the presence of fluorine, Churchill requested various water samples from McKay's research of areas with endemic mottling. With this research, Churchill and ALCOA reported that there were high fluoride levels, measured at 13.7 parts per million (ppm), in Bauxite's water supply (Mullen, 2005). Churchill also analyzed 26 samples from large cities within the United States and found less than 1.0ppm fluoride in all of them. Twenty-nine years after McKay began his research, Churchill concluded that fluoride was the cause of the stains and McKay published the findings in 1931 (McNeil, 1985).

Until this discovery was reported, the U.S. Public Health Service ignored McKay's pleas for assistance. Even so, once McKay published Churchill's research as evidence that fluoride was the stain-causing agent, the U.S. Public Health Service ordered the National Institutes of Health (NIH) to start government-sponsored dental research to verify the relationship between waterborne fluoride and the endemic mottling of teeth. Dr. H. Trendley Dean, the first director of the NIH, conducted an epidemiological study to confirm the correlation between fluoride levels and severe staining. The NIH first noted some communities had naturally higher levels of fluoride in their water and hoped for a solution to reduce these elevated levels. For this reason, several researchers started a project designing filters to adjust the levels of waterborne fluoride (Carstairs, 2015). Dean first published his systemic surveys in 1933, soliciting each state dental society for information on the occurrence and extent of the teeth mottling (McClure, 1970). In Dean's studies, McKay's

1916 report and other past research were used to develop standards of classification for mottled teeth. The water history of all the places Dean surveyed and the amount of fluoride in the water were thoroughly examined. Altogether, Dean and his associates established that fluoride levels up to 1.0ppm did not cause severe staining. This meant that discoloration of the tooth began when there were more than 1.0ppm fluoride in the water supply[10,11].

Furthermore, Dean surveyed the physiological effects of fluoride in drinking water and whether it caused dental cavities (McClure,1970). In addition to the endemic staining, the study of the physiological effects revealed a concomitant reduction in dental cavities. Gradually, this research led to further epidemiological studies establishing the relationship between water fluoridation and the reduction of dental cavities, and exposing the benefits of fluoride in water. In 1938, Dean published an article based on his research, showing children living in areas with fluoride of 1.0ppm had lower incidence of dental cavities compared to children without fluoride in their water (Carstairs, 2015). In 1942, Dean published additional research suggesting that the addition of artificial fluoride to community water supplies with natural fluoride levels lower than 1.0ppm was safe and effective for preventing dental cavities (Mullen, 2005). This led to effective community water fluoridation, which in turn predicated a decline in dental cavities during the second half of 20th century[11].

MILESTONE STUDIES

The Milestone studies were conducted by Bibley (1941) and Knutson (1942, 1947, 1948). These studies not only varied in concentration of NaF used but also in number of application / year.

1. **1941 Bibby– Ist clinical study-** 0.1% Nat was applied for 7-8min, 3 times in a year at 4 monthly interval in Ist year and 2 months interval in IInd year. The results showed 45% of reduction in caries in I year and 33% after 2 years and 36% at the end of 3rd year[12].

2. **Knutson and Armstrong (1942)-** In 1942 Knutson began a series of clinical trials (utilising 2% Nat solution for 3-4 minutes). Knutson concluded that maximum reduction in caries was achieved from 4 treatments at weekly intervals and suggested that the series of applications should be carried out at the ages of 3,7,10 and 13 years to coincide with the eruption of teeth. Gave 8-15 applications of Nat in the 1st year of a 3 year study. Percentage reduction was found to be : 39 8% after 1 year, 41.4% after 2 years 36.7% after 3 years[12].

3. **Knutson et al (1947)-** In 3 groups of 7-15 years children gave 2, 4 and 6 applications / year respectively and after 2 years found : 9.3% reduction in 1st group 20.1% in second group and 21% in 3rd group[12].

4. **Galgan and Knutson (1941)-** 3 groups of 7015 years children gave 2, 4 and 6 applications / year and the results after one year showed 21, 40.7 and 41.0% decrease caries respectively[12].

On the basis of above studies Knutson and Feldmand (1948) recommended a technique of 4 application of NaF at weekly intervals in a year and also recommended 3, 7, 10 and 13 years as specific age groups for NaF applications.

Many of the subsequent studies which have followed Knutsons techniques have shown DMFS decrease to the extent of 23.6% by Howell (1955) , 20% after 2 years by Jorell and Ericson (1965), 11% after 3 years by Cons et al (1970), 34% after 3 years by Swejda (1971)One disadvantage of the use of Knutson's technique is the patient must make 4 visits to the dentist with in a relatively short time. A few clinical trials on NaF done after 1965, authors have deviated from Knutson's technique by changing the weekly applications schedule to six monthly / yearly.Averilly et al (1967) tried 2 applications / year and found 11% fewer DMFS after 2 yearsMercer and Muhler (1972) found 27% fewer DMFS after one year by giving one application / year [12].

TOPICAL FLUORIDE:

"A fluoride applied directly to the teeth, especially of children, in a dental caries prevention program" (Miller-Keene & O'Toole, 2005).Topical fluorides are delivered to exposed surfaces of the dentition, at elevated concentrations for a local protective effect in making the teeth more resistant to decay.Topical fluorides are applied to the teeth directly and are most effective when delivered at very low doses several times a day (Ijaz, 2010). Topical treatments can be divided into self-applied and professionally applied fluorides. Self-applied therapy includes toothpastes and mouthrinses, while fluoride gels, foams, and varnishes are typically applied to teeth by a dental professional[13].

HOME APPLIED / SELF APPLIED

FLUORIDE DENTRIFICES:

Probably the most widespread and significant vehicle used for fluoride has been toothpastes. Introduced in the late 1960s and early 1970s, their rapid increase in market share was remarkable. The consensus view from developed countries was that the introduction of fluoride toothpaste was the single factor most responsible for the massive reduction in dental caries seen in many countries during the 1970s and 1980s[14].

Toothpaste has an important functions in maintaining oral health. It helps the consumers in the removal of plaque and debris by its detergent action. Polishing the tooth surface with toothpaste helps prevent the accumulation of microorganisms and debris. In modern life, toothpastes are used by individuals on a daily basis and hence can be a source of various therapeutic agents including F.29 Toothpastes containing F were first available commercially in the 1970s and are the major source of F in some communities where fluoridated drinking water is not available. F is added into toothpastes mostly as sodium fluoride (NaF), sodium monofluorophosphate (MFP), amine fluoride, and stannous fluoride[15]. The active ingredient in this toothpaste is sodium fluoride. This agent can be recommended for children 6 years and older and adolescents who are at high risk of caries and who are able to expectorate after brushing. Dentists may also prescribe this agent for adolescents who are undergoing orthodontic treatment, as they are at increased risk of caries during this time[16]. The other ingredients of toothpaste may also affect the availability of F in the oral cavity. Tooth brushing with fluoridated toothpaste is close to an ideal public health method in that its use is convenient, inexpensive, culturally approved and widespread [Burt, 1998][15,16].

This is especially true in the case of calcium containing abrasives due to their potential to inactivate the F. Similarly, F will react with silica to form fluorosilicates if a sufficient amount of detergent is not present. The use of fluoridated toothpastes has been demonstrated to have a caries reduction efficacy 25% greater than that for non-fluoridated tooth pastes. However, the benefits and therapeutic efficacy of using fluoridated tooth pastes may be affected by multiple factors such as the concentration of F, the amount of toothpaste used, and individual variations including the duration and frequency of brushing and rinsing behavior[17]. The main concern with this delivery method is inappropriate handling, particularly by children. The ingestion of fluoridated toothpastes can produce serious toxic effects and appropriate adult supervision is essential for children using toothpaste. Toothpastes are available in a wide range of F concentrations[18].

Toothpaste is a paste or gel dentifrice that is composed of water, abrasives, humectants, detergents, flavoring agents, antibacterial agents, and most important fluoride. Abrasives, which include calcium carbonate, dehydrated silica gels, hydrated aluminum oxides, magnesium carbonate, phosphate salts and silicates, are incorporated to remove food debris, plaque, and surface stains from teeth (Marinho, 2003). Another toothpaste ingredient is humectants, which include glycerol, xylitol, and sorbitol. Humectants are agents that prevent water loss in toothpaste and reduce the tendency of toothpaste to dry into a powder. Additionally, detergents in the toothpaste create a foaming action that helps with even toothpaste distribution, which improves cleansing power. These include sodium lauryl sulfate and sodium N-Lauryl sarcosinate. In order to encourage the use of toothpaste, flavoring agents, such as saccharin, are included in toothpaste for taste. These flavoring agents come in a variety of colors and flavors. Even though these flavoring agents are sweeteners, they do not promote tooth decay (Marinho, 2003). Understandably, antibacterial agents, such as Triclosan and zinc chloride, are also common ingredients in toothpaste. Their role is to prevent buildup of hardened plaque, also referred to as tartar. In addition these antibacterial agents can help reduce bad breath and gingivitis, a mild inflammation of gum tissue. Besides these ingredients, some toothpaste can consist of potassium nitrate or strontium chloride which helps in reducing tooth sensitivity[13].

Fluoride toothpaste has consistently been proven to provide a caries-preventive effect for individuals of all ages. In the United States, the fluoride concentration of over-the-counter toothpaste ranges from 1000 to 1100 ppm. In some other countries, toothpastes containing 1500 ppm of fluoride are available. A 1-inch (1-g) strip of toothpaste translates to 1 or 1.5 mg of fluoride, respectively. A pea-sized amount of toothpaste is approximately one-quarter of an inch. Therefore, a pea-sized amount of toothpaste containing 1000/1100 ppm of fluoride would have approximately 0.25 mg of fluoride, and the same amount of toothpaste containing 1500 ppm of fluoride would have approximately 0.38 mg of fluoride. Parents should supervise children younger than 8 years to ensure the proper amount of toothpaste and effective brushing technique. Children younger than 6 years are more likely to ingest some or all of the toothpaste used. Ingestion of excessive amounts of fluoride can increase the risk of fluorosis. This excess can be minimized by limiting the amount of toothpaste used and by storing toothpaste where young children cannot access it without parental help[16]. Use of fluoride toothpaste should begin with the eruption of the first tooth. When fluoride toothpaste is used for children younger than 3 years, it is recommended that the amount be limited to a smear or grain of rice size (about one-half of a pea). Once the child has turned 3 years of age, a pea-sized amount of toothpaste should be used[19]. Young children should not be given water to rinse after brushing because their instinct is to swallow. Expectorating without rinsing will both reduce the amount of fluoride swallowed and leave some fluoride in the saliva, where it is available for uptake by the dental plaque. Parents should be strongly advised to supervise their child's use of fluoride toothpaste to avoid overuse or ingestion. High-concentration toothpaste (5000 ppm) is available by prescription only[16].

Figure 2: Rice grain sized portion of toothpaste on a child's toothbrush on the left. A pea-sized portion of toothpaste on the right[20]

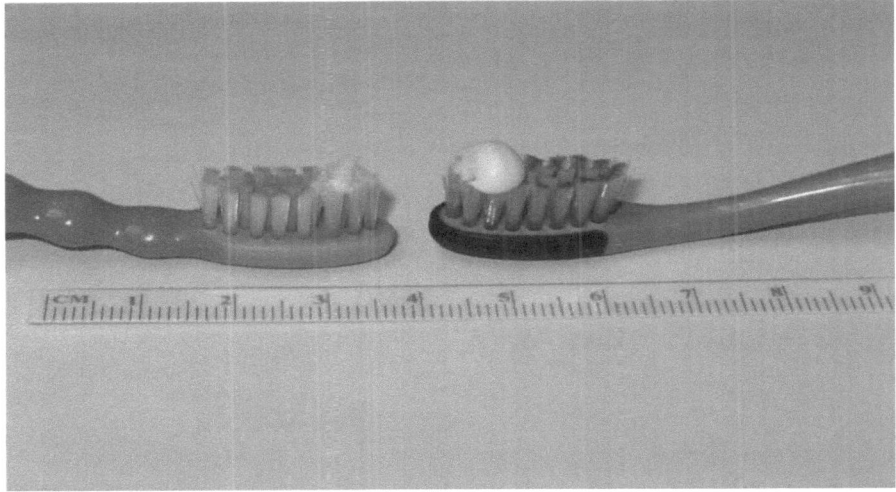

A rice grain sized portion of toothpaste on a child's toothbrush is shown on the left. A pea-sized portion of toothpaste is shown on the right[21].

Toothpaste tubes containing fluoride are now labeled and contain approximately 0.5 mg fluoride per gram of toothpaste. Some tubes suggest covering the bristles with toothpaste. A 'peasized' portion weighs approximately 0.75 g and contains about 0.4 mg of fluoride; a 'full cover' portion weighs approximately 2.25 g and contains about 1.0 mg of fluoride. Thus, brushing twice a day would deliver 0.8 to 2.0 mg of fluoride, depending on which regimen is used. If swallowed, the amount of fluoride could be excessive and could contribute to the development of fluorosis [22].

The duration of tooth brushing should exceed one minute on each occasion and children should be encouraged to spit out excess toothpaste and avoid rinsing with water. There is no firm evidence to suggest the ideal timing of tooth brushing but a common recommendation is that children's teeth should be brushed last thing at night before bedtime and on at least one other occasion. Eating directly after brushing should be avoided. Children's teeth can be brushed with either manual or powered toothbrushes with a soft small head[23].There are three categories of fluoride from toothpaste during tooth brushing: free ionic fluoride which has the ability to react with tooth structure, interfere with microbial metabolism, absorb to the oral mucosa, and has anticaries efficacy; profluoride compounds that are delivered or precipitate in the oral cavity during brushing, release ionic fluoride over time, and contribute to anticaries efficacy; and unavailable fluoride compounds that do not release fluoride ions, are either spat out or swallowed, and have no anticaries efficacy[24].

Composition of Fluoride Dentifrices

1. Abrasive Agents – The type of abrasive used in the fluoride dentifrice must be compatible with the fluoride agent used. The various type of abrasive agents used are Ca- pyrophosphate, Na- metaphospate , Silica

2. Fluoride Agents in Dentifrice- Types of fluoridated agents in dentifrices include;

1. Sodium fluoride (NaF).

2. Stannous fluoride (SnF2)

3. Sodium monofluorophosphate (MPF)

4. Amine fluoride

5. Combination of NaF and MPF[25]

   a. **Sodium monofluorophosphate Dentifrices-** Dentifrices containing 850 to 1,150 ppm theoretical total fluorine in a gel or paste dosage form. Sodium monofluorophosphate 0.654 to 0.884% with an available fluoride ion concentration (consisting of PO3F= and F- combined) = 800 ppm. Dentifrices containing 1,500 ppm theoretical total fluorine in a gel or paste dosage form. Sodium monofluorophosphate 1.153% with an available fluoride ion concentration = 1,275 ppm.

b. **Stannous fluoride Dentifrices-** Dentifrices containing 850 to 1,150 ppm theoretical total fluorine in a gel or paste dosage form. Stannous fluoride 0.351 to 0.474% with an available fluoride ion concentration = 700 ppm for products containing abrasives other than calcium pyrophosphate. Stannous fluoride 0.351 to 0.474% with an available fluoride ion concentration = 290 ppm for products containing the abrasive calcium pyrophosphate[26].

c. **Sodium fluoride Dentifrices-** Dentifrices containing 350 to 1,150 ppm theoretical total fluorine in a gel or paste dosage form. Sodium fluoride 0.188 to 0.254% with an available fluoride ion concentration = 650 ppm. Sodium fluoride 0.188 to 0.254% with an available fluoride ion concentration of = 850 ppm for products containing the abrasive sodium bicarbonate and a poured-bulk density of 1.0 to 1.2 g/ml.[1472] The range of fluoride concentrations in these agents is 525 – 1450 ppm. The content of fluoride in dentifrices will decrease with the increase in the time of storage i.e six months or more[26].

d. **Amine fluoride or ammonium fluoride.** - In 1957, Muhlemann and coworkers of the university of Zurich, first studied the effects of amine fluorides on enamel solubility in vitro. Under the conditions of their study, certain organic fluorides were superior to inorganic fluoride in reducing enamel solubility. They attributed the improved effect to a combination of chemical protection afforded by the fluoride and physico chemical protection due to the organic portion of the molecule. In addition to their ability to reduce enamel solubility, the amine fluorides have other properties that enhance their potential cariostatic agents. Some of them are surface active that is they have an affinity for enamel and thus will hold fluoride for longer time against the tooth.

Amine fluoride preparations contain a mixture of 2 long chains – aliphatic amine hydrofluorides at pH-4.5. Reduction of enamel solubility from amine fluoride was reported to be better than SnF_2 and APF. Fluoride deposition occurs primarily by formation of CaF_2. However CaF_2 precipitates formed on the enamel surface are different from those formed by NaF possibly because of adsorption of amine moiety. Amine portion of this agent has both surfactant and antimicrobial properties.

e. **Stannous Hexfuorozirconate [SnZrF$_6$]-** Researchers at Indian University have developed a new compound, stannous hexafluorozirconate which according to invitro and invivo studies are said to be effective in reducing the solubility of enamel and in preventing dental caries. However the number and magnitude of negative incremental caries scores are disconcerting of results of 2 preliminary studies with children receiving semiannual applications of stannous hexaflurozirconate. The FDA has requested of the sponsor that no further studies he instituted until adequate pre-clinical studies have been performed to demonstrate safety.

f. **Monofluorophosphate-** Sodium monofluorophosphate differs from all other agents used for topical fluoride therapy Fluoride atom is covalently bonded to a phosphorous atom. It is also unique because only fluorapatite forms even when it is applied to enamel in high concentration or at low pH. The mechanisms include direct incorporation of the PO$_3$F^{2-} anion (MFP) into Hap / first it hydrolyses to phosphate and fluoride ions, which then react to form FA.

$$PO_3F^{2-} + OH^- \longrightarrow PO_4^{2-} + F^- + H^+$$

It has been proposed that MFP is initially acquired intact by enamel. During caries attack it is released and hydrolysed to fluoride ions, which then reacts to form FA. Hydrolysis of MFP is also catalysed by salivary enzymes. Because plaque can accumulate MFP, it can serve as a depot where slow hydrolysis can occur, thus slowly releasing fluoride ions to react with enamel. When pH is lowered during a caries attack, the rate of hydrolysis is increased at a time when fluoride is best utilized. Sodium MFP has been tested in professionally applied fluoride preventive programs, it has been never marketed as such[26].

Factors Affecting Dentifrice Effectiveness

In addition to the inherent properties of a fluoride dentifrice product, biological and behavioral factors can modify its anticaries effectiveness. All of these factors interplay in what can be described as the "application" phase (the initial interaction of relatively high concentrations of fluoride with the tooth surface and plaque), and the "retention" phase (the fluoride remaining in the mouth after brushing that is retained in saliva, plaque and plaque fluid, the tooth surface, and oral soft tissue reservoirs)[27]. Behavioral factors include the frequency of dentifrice use, length of brushing, rinsing practices after brushing, the time of day that dentifrice is applied, and amount of dentifrice applied to the brush. It is well established that the frequency of use has a major influence on effectiveness. Bushing twice per day or more has a greater preventive effect than once per day [28]. Length of the brushing time (application phase) determines how long the relatively high fluoride concentration in the dentifrice slurry stays in contact with the teeth and plaque, allowing fluoride uptake to take place. The higher the fluoride concentration, the greater the driving force for fluoride diffusion through plaque toward the tooth surface. Rinsing behaviors after toothbrushing affect the amount of fluoride retained in the mouth and have been reported to affect caries experience. Physiologic (biological) factors, mainly salivary flow rate during and after fluoride application influence the rate of fluoride clearance[29]. Bedtime use of fluoride dentifrice results in longer fluoride retention than daytime application due to greatly decrease salivary flow during sleep. The amount of fluoride applied to the toothbrush (dose) is not as important as the concentration of available fluoride in a dentifrice. Reduced fluoride concentration dentifrices are not as effective as regular concentration products. The fluoride dose is, however, important in regard to enamel fluorosis in children under six years of age because of dentifrice ingestion. For this reason, reducing the amount of fluoride applied is a better strategy than lowering the dose of products intended for use by children[28].

Recommendations for Use of Fluoride Dentifrice

The following recommendations are offered for the use of fluoride-containing dentifrices:

1. Oral cleanings after feedings should begin prior to primary tooth eruption, but certainly as soon as teeth have erupted. Nonfluoride, all-natural tooth cleaning gels are available for use in low-caries-risk children at this age Because of the association between fluorosis and fluoride toothpaste use in children younger than 2, use of fluoridated dentifrices prior to age 2 should be based on a caries risk assessment. Parents should be apprised of the risks and benefits of fluoride dentifrice use in this age group.

2. Tooth-brushing should be supervised by an adult, especially once fluoride dentifrice use has begun. Pea-sized dabs of dentifrice should be used, and the caregiver should brush the child's teeth until this is no longer practicable. At that point, the parent should continue to dispense the dentifrice and the child should have his tooth-brushing checked by the caregiver.

3. Tooth-brushing with a fluoridated toothpaste should be done twice daily. This frequency is associated with additional benefits over once-daily brushing, but the benefits of more frequent cleanings are not well established.

4. Older children who are able to expectorate should use more than a pea-sized dab to increase their salivary fluoride levels[30].

5. In Children under five years: - A brush full of 1000-ppm paste may contain (1 mg F ions). Child may swallow pastes accidentally, at this age the child cannot control muscles of swallowing. Thus brushing twice a day with 1000 ppm fluoridated paste the child may swallow 0.5 mg F/day. The child may be at risk to be affected by dental fluorosis, especially in fluoridated area or taking fluoride supplements.

6. In Children above 5 – years and adults - For children, in fluoridated and non-fluoridated area a high concentration of fluoride can be used[25].

7. The ingestion of more than the recommended daily dose of fluoride is associated with an increased risk of dental fluorosis .

8. In the absence of adequate topical fluoride exposure (eg, fluoridated toothpaste or water), additional fluoride products may be provided in the form of drops, chewable tablets and lozenges. The effectiveness of these products in preventing dental caries is low in school-aged children and has not been evaluated in infants and toddlers.

9. The EAPD recommendations for the use of fluoride toothpaste in children are summarized in below. The daily use of fluoride toothpaste, in combination with oral hygiene instructions, is recommended as the basic part of a caries-preventive program in addition to other caries-preventive methods, such as diet counselling, topical use of fluorides and fissure sealants, which are also important. [23]

Figure 3: Recommended use of fluoride toothpaste in children[23]

Age Group	Fluoride concentration	Daily use	Amount to be used
6 months- <2 years	500 ppm	twice	pea-size
2-<6 Years	1000 (+)ppm	twice	pea-size
6 years and over	1450 ppm	twice	1-2 cm

FLUORIDE MOUTHRINSES

It was started in the early 60,s of the last century[25]. Mouth washes can be used in conjunction with toothpaste and are recommended for patients with a high susceptibility to dental caries. The active compound for F delivery in mouth rinses is sodium fluoride (NaF). Commonly available over the counter mouth rinses contain 0.05% NaF (equivalent to 226 ppm of F)[31]. F-containing mouth rinses have the advantage of having a lower viscosity than toothpastes which allows the F to reach into difficult to access areas such as the interproximal regions, narrow pits, and fissures. F delivery through a mouth rinse is recommended for children over 6 years with active dental caries, patients undergoing fixed orthodontic treatment to reduce the chances of demineralization around orthodontic brackets, patients with decreased salivary flow, and patients with decreased manual dexterity[32]. In order to prevent its ingestion, mouthwashes must not be prescribed for children under 6 years of age and mentally retarded patients[19]. A mechanistic perspective, fluoride mouthrinses can lead to higher levels of oral fluoride retention than fluoride dentifrice, depending on behavioral practices after tooth brushing[26].

Mouthrinses are generally composed of water, alcohol, cleansing agents, and flavoring and coloring agents (Marinho, 2003). Cleansings agents include fluoride, astringent salts, antimicrobial agents, and odor neutralizers (Marinho, 2003). Fluoride helps reduce small carious lesions on tooth enamel and acts to make teeth more resistant to decay. Antimicrobial agents are included in rinses in order to help reduce plaque and gingivitis, as well as controlling bad breath. Astringent salts are incorporated to serve as deodorizers and to reduce bad breath, while odor neutralizers work to inactivate odor causing compounds. Mouthwashes can be categorized as cosmetic or therapeutic. Cosmetic rinses can temporarily reduce bad breath, but do not actually eliminate the odor causing bacteria (Marinho, 2003). In addition cosmetic mouthwashes do not help reduce plaque, gingivitis, or cavities. On the other hand, therapeutic mouthwashes are able to reduce plaque, gingivitis, cavities and bad breath. Therapeutic rinses specifically contain fluoride which helps prevent or reduce tooth decay. Furthermore, therapeutic mouthwashes act directly on bacteria present in plaque, which does not allow plaque to accumulate and progress to the early stages of gingivitis (Marinho, 2003). Antimicrobial agents found in therapeutic rinses help to eliminate bad breath and inactivate odor causing compounds[13].

Fluoride mouthrinses have been available for several decades in the United States as solutions containing:

1. .05% NaF (~226 ppm F) or acidulated phosphate fluoride (APF) for daily use; or

2. .2% NaF (~900 ppm F) solutions for weekly use.

Both concentrations were originally available as prescription-only ingestible solutions, with the .2% formulations reserved primarily for school-based mouthrinse programs. In the 1980s, the FDA permitted the marketing of over-the-counter .05% NaF solutions that were not intended for ingestion[25].

The use of mouthrinses to deliver chemotherapeutic agents is well accepted by the public, both by self administration and under supervision, mainly in school fluoride rinsing programs[33]. School based fluoride mouth rinse (FMR) programs were introduced in the 1970s to reduce the prevalence of caries in children (Divaris, 2012). The school setting was deemed as a favorable environment for a caries prevention program because it could more effectively treat those children who come from a disadvantaged background and experience a higher incidence of dental caries due to lack of access to oral healthcare or financial restraints (Divaris, 2012). Generally the schedule for school based FMR programs is a supervised weekly administration of 10 ml of a mouthwash containing .20% sodium fluoride that 27 students vigorously rinse for 60 seconds (ASTDD, 2012). For use at home, over the counter fluoride mouthwashes, which contain only .05% sodium fluoride, can be used for daily rinsing (ASTDD, 2012)[13].

Mouthrinse formulations are generally much simpler than dentifrices, and compatibility problems are not as large an issue as they are with dentifrice products. While mouthrinses are a heavily utilized oral care vehicle with over 120 million mouthwash users in the US, fluoride mouthrinses represent only 7% of the total mouthrinse business in the US, and thus, there is considerable room for increasing use of this approach for delivering fluoride. Many types of mouthrinse active ingredients have been evaluated for their plaque-reducing effectiveness and ability to reduce mutans streptococci, including chlorhexidine, essential oils, triclosan, cetylpyridinium chloride, sanquinarin, sodium dodecyl sulphate, and various metal ions (tin, zinc, copper). However, the evidence supporting the effectiveness of antiplaque agents in preventing dental caries, with the possible exception of chlorhexidine, is very limited; therefore, fluoride-containing mouthrinse will be the main focus here[34].

Fluoride mouthrinses may have a caries-protective effect in children with limited exposure to other sources of fluoride, but that any additional effect is questionable in children who use a fluoridated dentifrice daily. There was insufficient evidence to permit an analysis of the effectiveness of fluoride mouthrinse in the primary dentition[30].

Uses of Fluoride Mouthrinses

 a) Primary preventive programs for children and adults

 b) In subjects with high risk to dental caries.

 c) Patients with rampant caries.

 d) Patients with hyposalivations or xerostomia.

 e) Patients with sensitive teeth due to tooth wear as (abrasion, attrition, erosion) or because of exposed root

 f) Patients with periodontits and root caries.

 g) Patients with orthodontic appliance[25].

 h) Patients those wearing intraoral prostheses[30].

Types of agents used:

1. **Sodium fluoride**: It is the main type used in neutral or acidified forms in a water vehicle.
 Concentrations: 0.2% (900 ppm F) applied once a week.
        0.05% (225 ppm) applied daily.

2. **Stannous fluoride** :Concentration 100, 200, 300 ppm[25].

Fluoridated mouth rinse should not be given

1. To children under six years of age, as they cannot control muscles of swallowing. As with fluoridated dentifrices, swallowing of fluoride mouthrinses is an issue for children who have not yet mastered their swallowing reflex. Therefore, these products should be recommended for only those children who demonstrate the ability to swish and expectorate without swallowing (generally age 6 or older).

2. Children living in fluoridated area or receiving fluoride supplements. Fluoridated mouth rinses should not substitute fluoridated dentifrices, rinses is usually supplement toothpaste[25].

Recommendations for Use of Fluoride Mouthrinse

Based on the current literature regarding fluoride mouthrinses, the following recommendations are offered:

1. Fluoride mouthrinses should be reserved for use with children judged to be at moderate or high risk for dental caries, including children with fixed orthodontic or prosthetic appliances and those with reduced salivary flow.

2. Daily use of an over-the-counter .05% NaF rinse in a swish-and-expectorate regimen is as effective as a prescription rinse that is swallowed after rinsing.

3. Little additional benefit should be expected from fluoride mouthrinses in low-caries-risk children who are already using a fluoridated dentifrice.

4. Fluoride mouthrinses should be recommended only for those children who have demonstrated mastery of their swallowing reflex.

5. Where available, alcohol-free preparations should be recommended over those containing alcohol[30].

TOPICAL FLUORIDE FOAM :

In 1993, Sodium Fluoride (NaF) foams were introduced to the United States market. These fluoride foams only underwent a short evolution and include acidulated phosphate foam (APF) for deep infiltration, and neutral fluoride foam for restorations or individuals sensitive to acidic fluorides. Neutral foams provide fluoride without damage to the surface of restorations and are a good alternative for acid-sensitive patients. Indications for fluoride foams are similar to other topical fluorides (i.e., desensitization and cavity prevention), but they are most effective in primary teeth and on the proximal surfaces. Recommended mainly for children, one study states that all ages can benefit from a 4-minute application of fluoride foam instead of a gel, since the foams are equally effective[35]. These foams have been marketed as "minute-foams," but just as with gels, a minimum 4-minute contact is recommended for adequate fluoride infiltration. Examples of neutral foams available are Topex Neutral Fluoride Foam (Sultan Healthcare, Inc. Hackensack, NJ) and Kolorz Neutral Fluoride Foam (DMG America, Englewood, NJ). Acidulated phosphate fluoride foam is available in products like Denti-Foam Topical Fluoride Foam (Medicom USA, Augusta, CA). These foams claim deeper fluoride infiltration and lengthier fluoride retention in saliva after treatment. Foams provide an average 25% caries reduction rate in adolescents and adults with moderate-to-high-risk for caries. Since foams are most effective on primary teeth, these rates can be much higher—up to 41%—in the children in moderate-to high - risk populations[36].

Advantages:

a. Requires smaller amount of application resulting in a lower fluoride dose

b. Better tolerated than gels (reduced gagging)

c. The weight of the clinical evidence of foam's effectiveness is not as strong as it is for fluoride gel/varnish[37].

SELF-APPLIED FLUORIDE GELS

Self-applied fluoride gels were originally developed for application via custom mouth trays, though no single application regimen has been considered standard. Fluoride gels are currently available by prescription for self-application as APF and neutral NaF products containing 1.1% NaF (5,000 ppm F ion). Some manufacturers have reformulated their NaF gels with abrasives as a reflection of the increasing use of these products in a brush-on regimen. Glycerin-based SnF_2 products (not true gels) are available with a concentration of 1,000 ppm F^{30}. Some gels and foams can be self-applied at home with the aid of a toothbrush, but the concentration of fluoride in these products is significantly lower. A dentist can also make a tray that is custom fitted for a patient's teeth, and fluoride treatments can be loaded into this tray and be used overnight at home[13].

Most studies of self-applied fluoride gel were conducted in the 1960s and 1970s with NaF or APF containing F concentrations of 5,000 or 12,300 ppm. Application frequencies ranged from 3 to 4 times per week during the school year to 4 times per calendar year. The percent of DMFS reductions in fluoride-deficient communities by tray application and brushing ranged from 0.5% to 80%, with a pooled average of approximately 32%. The dramatic reductions (80%) obtained by Englander et al (1967) in a nonfluoridated area have not been replicated in other studies. Caries reductions in trials conducted in optimally fluoridated communities ranged from 7% to 35%[38]. There are no well-designed clinical trials of SnF_2 gels. No systematic reviews of purely self-applied gels have been conducted.

Fluoride gels and pastes are often recommended by practitioners for patients:

1. With severe early childhood caries;

3. With rampant caries in the mixed and permanent dentitions;

4. With reduced salivary flow;

5. Wearing prosthetic or orthodontic appliances; and

6. Who may be at high risk for dental caries[30].

Recommendations for the use

1. These products should be recommended for patients in fluoride-deficient communities who are at high risk for caries.

2. Parents of young children should supervise placement of the product in the custom tray or on the toothbrush. In a brush-on technique with young children, only a pea-sized amount should be used. Brushing should be supervised and, preferably, done by an adult. In tray applications, only the minimum amount of gel necessary to cover the teeth should be used. Tray application should not exceed 4 minutes. Patients should be cautioned against swallowing the gel, and should be allowed to expectorate freely after either type of application. Rinsing, eating, and drinking should be delayed for 30 minutes. Ideally, gel application should occur just prior to bedtime. Caution is advised regarding the use of prescription fluoride gels and pastes in children younger than 6 years.

3. Application regimens should be limited to the minimum time period deemed necessary for control of dental caries, and patients should be evaluated periodically to determine when self-application can be terminated[30].

PROFESSIONALLY APPLIED

Professional topical fluorides include fluoride gels, foams, rinses and varnishes. Traditionally, professional fluoride treatment in the US and Canada involved the use of fluoride gels in trays. This was followed by the introduction of fluoride foams used in trays, which are generally considered easier to use than gels and have less risk of ingestion of fluoride. Less total fluoride is applied with foam, and a lower volume of product is used. These factors reduce the risk of the patient gagging and swallowing fluoride and also the amount of fluoride that could be ingested as a result. Fluoride varnish has been in use in Europe for more than 30 years as a method of professional application of topical fluoride[39]. In North America, sodium fluoride varnish was introduced first in Canada, and later in the US when it was cleared by the Food and Drug Administration (FDA) for use as a desensitizing agent and cavity liner. As such, its use for caries prevention in the US is "off-label" (i.e., it is being used for a purpose that has not received FDA approval or clearance). Since its introduction in the United States in the 1990s, its use for the prevention of caries has increased among the dental community[40].

Fluoride gels and foams are generally administered by a dentist for patients who are at high risk for dental caries. For individuals at a moderate risk for caries, fluoride gels or foams are recommended every 6 months (Marinho, 2002). High risk individuals can receive gel treatments as often as every 3 months (Marinho, 2002). In a professional setting, a dentist will load the gel or foam into a tray then insert it into the patient's mouth. Approximately 5 ml of gel is used in a single tray (Marinho, 2002). The patient bites down on the tray for about four minutes. Afterwards, patients are advised not to rinse, eat, or drink for about 30 minutes in order to prolong contact between the fluoride and tooth enamel. Fluoride gels do contain abrasives, such as calcium carbonate, dehydrated silica gels, hydrated aluminum oxides, magnesium carbonate, phosphate salts and silicates, which can be found in toothpaste (Marinho, 2002). The concentration of fluoride in gels is significantly higher than that which is found in toothpaste. Fluoride gels can include sodium fluoride, stannous fluoride and acidulated phosphate fluoride. Typically, gels will consist of 12,300 ppm F (Marinho, 2002). Because this is such a highly concentrated form of fluoride, excessive ingestion of gels can lead to acute toxicity. Nausea, vomiting, headache and abdominal pain are symptoms if overexposure of fluoride occurs (Marinho, 2002). Because of the risk of over ingestion the use of gels in young children is not recommended (Marinho, 2002)[13].

Concentration:

a. 2% Sodium Fluoride (NaF)

b. 8% Stannous Fluoride (SnF2)

c. Acidulated Phosphate Fluoride (APF) with 1.23% fluoride.

d. Fluoride Varnish

e. Prophylactic Paste[37]

SODIUM FLUORIDE-

Neutral sodium fluoride was the first topically applied agent studied independently by Knutson and Armstrong (1943) and Bibby (1944). A 2% NaF solution was applied topically in series of four treatments at intervals of about one week at ages 3, 7, 10, and 13, at times when various groups of primary and permanent teeth usually erupt (Knutson and Armstrong, 1943). These procedures were time-consuming and did not coincide with regular dental check-ups. Therefore, in Scandinavia, sodium fluoride solutions have usually been applied from one to four times per year. Recently, 2% NaF gels have been marketed[41].

Methods of preparation of 2%NaF:

2%Naf solution can be prepared by dissolving 20gms of Naf powder in 1 lt of distilled water in a plastic bottle. It is essential to store F(Fluoride) in plastic bottles because it stored in glass containers, the fluoride ion of solution can react with silica of glass forming SiF2, thus reducing the availability of free active F for anticaries action[12].

Method of application of NaF according to Knuston technique

Initially cleaning and polishing of the teeth is done in only the 1st of the four application an upper and opposing lower quadrant are opposing lower quadrants are isolated with cotton rolls and the teeth are dried thoroughly.

2% NaF is then applied with cotton applicators and is permitted to dry on the teeth for about 4 minutes. The procedure is repeated for the remaining quadrants. After completion of the treatment the patient is instructed to avoid eating, drinking or rinsing for 30 min so as to prolong the availability of fluoride ion to react with the tooth surfaces. $2^{nd}, 3^{rd}, 4^{th}$ application are given at weekly intervals. A full series of four treatments is recommended at ages 3,7,11 and 13[12].

Mechanism of action of NaF

When NaF is applied topically, it reacts with hydroxyapetite crystals to form CaF_2 which is the dominant product of reaction.

$$Ca(PO_4)_6 (OH)_2 + 20F \rightleftharpoons 10CaF_2 + 6HPO_4^{3-} + 2(OH)^-$$

This is due to conc. Of F in 2%NaF due to which the solubility product of CaF_2 get exceeded fast and this initial rapid reaction is followed by drastic reduction in its rate and the phenomenon is called choking off. This occurs because once a thick layer of CaF_2 get formed it interfers with further diffusion of F from the topical F solution to react with hydroxyapetite to form fluoridated hydroxyapetite.

$$CaF_2 + 2Ca_5 (PO_4)_3 OH \rightleftharpoons 2Ca_5 (PO_4)_3 F + Ca(OH)_2$$

which increase the concentration of surface fluoride thus making the tooth structure more metabolism through anti-enzymatic action and also helps in remineralization of the initial decalcified areas thus showing its manifold anticaries effect[12].

Advantages

a) It is relatively stable when kept in a plastic container and there is no need to prepare a fresh solution for each patient.

b) The taste is well accepted by patients. The solution is non-irritating to the gingival and does not cause discoloration of tooth structure.

c) Once applied to the teeth, the solution is allowed to dry for 3 minutes, thus the clinician in public health programs can pursue a multiple chair procedures.

d) The series of treatments must be repeated only 4 times in the general age range of 3-17, rather than at annual or semiannual intervals[12].

Disadvantages

The major disadvantage of the use of sodium fluoride is that the patient must make 4 visits to the dentist within a relatively short time[12].

ACIDULATED PHOSPHATE FLUORIDE

APF was introduced in the 1960's(Brudevolde?a/., 1963) and is available in solutions and gels. These agents contain 1.23% fluoride in the form of sodium fluoride at pH 3.0. At this pH, more than 50% of the fluoride will be in the form of HF rather than as free fluoride ions. Phosphate was added to an acid fluoride solution to depress calcium fluoride formation and increase fluorapatite formation. Several studies have shown that even APF agents produce substantial amounts of calcium fuoride (Bruun et al., 1983b; Retief et ai, 1983). APF is generally applied at six- or 12-month intervals and has become more popular than sodium fluoride solutions. APF gels are applied in mouth trays, are more convenient to apply, and require less chair-time than solutions. APF gels are the most widely used preparation for topical application in the USA. The use of APF in Europe is limited[41].

APF has been used at the countries with high caries activites, low consciousness level in prevention, and the system of dental health treatment that is not well organized yet. APF is sodium fluoride derivate in the form of solution, gel or powder which characterizes acid at pH 3 to 4 and characterizes buffer f it interacts with phosphate. APF has been tested in its use, both in the form of solution or gel, but gel is the form which is most frequently used. This agent has better ability in bonding to enamel calcium. It also non irritating and non staining that can be tolerated by adding the taste as well as easily accepted by patients. The affectivity of APF can be various, depends on the methods and frequency of its application[42]. This agent is a mineral which can strengthen the enamel surfaces and prevent root caries as well as inhibit caries risks as the effect of saliva product which is less because of radiation therapy or chemotherapy.

APF usually contains 2% sodium fluoride, 0.34% hydrogen fluoride and 0.98% phosphate acid.APF can be used for children 6 years up and adults with high caries risks but has contraindication to the patients who have hypersensitive reaction, the patients who have dental implant, patients with composite restoration, porcelain, compomer, and ionomer glass[43].

Methods of preparation of APF solution/ gel

Acidulated phosphate fluoride usually contains 1.23% fluoride(F) in o.1 M Phoshoric acid at a pH of 3.0 and is stable with long self life when stored in in opaque plastic bottles. It is prepared by dissolving 20 gm of NaF in 1 lt of 0.1 M Phosphoric acid. To this is added 50% Hydrofluoride acid to adjust the pH at 3.0 and f- concentration at 1.23%. For the preparation of APF gel a gallic agent Methycellulose or Hydroxyethyl cellulose is to be added to the solution and the pH is to be adjust between 4-5[12].

Method of application of APF

After thorough prophylaxis the teeth are isolated with cotton rolls on both lingual and buccal sides, dried and APF solution is continuosly and repeatedly applied with cotton applicators and the teeth are kept moist for 4 min. Floss may be drawn through each inter-proximal embrasures to ensure wetting to these surfaces. The recommended frequency of APF topical application is semi annually.

APF gel may be applied in the same manner as topical solution but APF gel can be used by self application procedure and children can be trained for this. A variety of self reusable/disposable tray in various size together with sponge like tray-liners are available[12].

Mechanism of action

Aasenden & Brudevold and McCann in 1968 reported that the tooth enamel acquired larger amount of F with deeper penetration when pretreated with dilute phosphoric acid before being exposed to F solution, Chow & Brown explained this deeper F penetration on the basis of formation of an intermediate product which was less stable and highly reactive with F as compared to Hap crystals. The authors further reported that when APF is applied on the teeth it initially leads to dehydration and shrinkage in the volume of Hap crystal which further on hydrolysis form an intermediate product called Dicalcium phosphate dehydrate(DCPD). This DCPD which is highly reactive with F Starts forming immediately forming APF is applied and F penetrates into the crystal more deeply through the opening produced by shrinkage and leads to formation of FA.

$$Ca_5(PO_4)_3OH + 4H^+ \rightleftharpoons 5Ca^{++} + CHPO_4^- + H_2O$$

$$Ca^{++} + HPO_4^{2-} \xrightleftharpoons{OH^-} Ca.HPO_4.2H_2O$$

$$5CaHPO_4.2H_2O \xrightleftharpoons{F^-} Ca_5(PO_4)_3F + 2HPO_4^{2-}$$

The amount and depth of F deposits as FAP would be dependent on the amount and depth which DCPD gets formed. Since for the conversion of whole of DCPD of formed into FAP deeper penetration and continuous supply of F is required so APF has to be applied every 30 sec and the teeth be kept wet for 4 min[12].

Advantages

a) Requires only 2 applications in a year and is thus suited for most dental office routines.

b) The gel can be self applied and thus the cost of application also gets reduced.

Disadvantages

a) Practical difficulties like the teeth should be kept wet for 4 min. So repeated applications necessitates, the use of solution thereby minimizing its use in the field. This also increases chair side time making this fluoride application program more expensive.

b) It is acidic and sour and bitter in taste.

c) It cannot be stored in glass containers. Because it may remove mineral from (etching) of the glass.

d) APF causes surface alternations of many restorative materials essentially degradation of the material[12].

STANNOUS FLUORIDE

After the discovery of NaF, a wide variety of other fluoride compounds were tried. E.g. : Potassium, lead, silicon, tin, zirconium. SnF_2 was found to be the most effective (Muller and Van Huysea, 1947). Muller et al in 1947 observed the enamel powders treated with stannous fluoride solution greatly reduced the rate of acid dissolution and in another in-vitro study (1950) found SnF_2 to be 3 times more effective than NaF. Much of the voluminous literature in 1950-60's deals with the relative efficacy of 2% NaF and SnF in varying concentrations of 2%, 8% and 10%. The first clinical trial utilizing 2% SnF_2 was carried out by, Howell and Muller - 1950 – studied relative efficacy of 4 applications of 2% SnF_2 and 2%. NaF reported 83% and 23.6% reduction in caries rate respectively while Nevitte et al., in the same year reported 44.4% reduction with SnF_2 and 35.9% with NaF. Since four applications 1 year as studied so far is not possible from public health point of view. Gish and Muller (1957) tried single annual application of (8% SnF_2) and compared with Knutson's technique of NaF application and reported SnF_2 to be 21% more effective than NaF after first year 32 and 35% after 2nd and 3rd years[16].

In the same year another study was done by Jorden et al in 12-15 years old children reported 20% and 38% reduction in caries rate at the end of 1st year and 2nd year of study respectively utilizing single annual application of 8% SnF_2.

Hauwink et al (1974) – longest clinical trial extending over a period of 9 years and utilizing 8% SnF_2 in 22 pairs of monozygotic twins, showed 37% caries reduction. The effect of 9 years treatment still apparent 5 years after treatment had stopped.

Stannous fluoride solutions and gels containing 8% or 10% fluoride and amine fluoride solutions and gels containing 1.0- 1.25% fluoride are also available for professional topical application. Stannous fluoride has a significant inhibiting effect on plaque acidogenicity (Svatun and Attramadal, 1978) and plaque formation (Svatun et al., 1977; Tinanoff, 1985). These effects are due to the stannous ion rather than the fluoride ion. Mild staining of teeth and an unpleasant taste have limited the clinical use of stannous fluoride. Also, amine fluoride has been reported to have a stronger antibacterial effect than most fluoride compounds (Gehring, 1981;Meurman, 1987)[12].

Method of preparation of Stannous fluoride

Stannous fluoride solution has to be freshly prepared before use each time as it no self life. For convention preparation 'O' no. Gelation capsules are priorly filled with 0.8 gm powered SnF2 and are stored in air tight plastic container. Just before application, the contain of one capsule is dissolved in 10 ml of distill water in plastic container and the solution thus prepared is shaken briefly.

The solution is applied immediately to the teeth. The 10 ml of solution should sufficient to treat the whole mouth of a single patient if any remains it should discarded and not used again.

Method of application of Stannous fluoride

The recommended procedure of topical application of SnF2 being with thorough prophylaxis. each tooth surface must be thoroughly cleaned and polished with pumice including the promimal surface. The teeth are then isolated with cotton roll and dried preferably with compressed air. Either a quadrant or half of the mouth can be treated at one time. Quadrant to be treated should be kept free of saliva and if possible a saliva ejector should be used. A freshly prepared 8% solution of stannous fluoride is applied continuously to the teeth with cotton applicator so that the teeth are kept moist with the solution for 4 min and a replication of solution to a particular tooth is done every 15-30 sec. The recommended frequency of 8% SnF2 application is one per year[12]

Mechanism of action of SnF2

Muhler(1968) reported that when SnF2 reacts with hydroxyapetite in addition of F the tin of SnF2 also react with enamel and a new crystal line product (Wei and forbes 1968) gets formed which is different from Flourapatite and this new compound which is Sn3F3Po4 is more resistant to decay then enamel(it is due to this reason that always a freshly prepared SnF2 solution should be used and the capsules of SnF2 should be kept in air tight container otherwise the Stannous form of tin gets oxydised to stannic form, thus making the Snf2 inactive for anticarious action). Infra redabsorption and X-ray diffraction analysis of a reaction of SnF2 with HA shows that mainly four and product get formed, tin Sn2(OH)PO4 is formed when SnF2 is applied in low conc. and the second the main end product which gets formed is Tin-Tri-FLourophoshate at very high concentration of SnF2 (Snf3)2) gets formed along with Sn3F3PO4(TTFP). CaF2 in low quantity is also te end product both in low and high concentration .

At low concentration

$$Ca_5(PO_4)_3OH + 2SnF_2 \longrightarrow 2CaF_2 + Sn_2(OH)(PO_4) + Ca_3(PO_4)_3$$

Tin hydroxy phosphate

At high concentration

$$Ca_5(PO_4)_3OH + 162SnF_2 \longrightarrow CaF_2 + Sn_2F_3PO_4 + Sn_2(OH)(PO_4) + 4CaF_2(SnF_3)_2$$

Tin trifluoro   Tinhydroxy   calcium

Phosphate   phosphate   trifluorostanate

CaF2 so formed further reacts with HA and small fractions of Flour-hydroxyapetite also get formed.

$$2Ca_5(PO_4)_3OH + CaF_2 \longrightarrow 2Ca_5(PO_4)_3F + Ca(OH)_2$$

The other end product,Tin hyrdroxyphosphate gets dissolved in oral fluids and is responsible for the metallic taste after opical application of SnF2. The main end product i.e Tin-Tri-fluorophosphate is responsible for making the tooth structure more stable and less susceptible to decay however recently Babcock et.al 1978 reported that Ca Tri-Fluorostannate has also got similar properties.

Advantages

The procedure frequency complies with one year recall appointment schedule.

Disadvantages

a) In aqueous solution the material is not stable undergoes fairly rapid hydrolysis and oxidation and forms a $Sn(OH)_2$ and stannic ion. This reaction reduces the agents' effectiveness. Consequently a fresh solution must be prepared for each treatment.

b) Since 8% solution is quite astringent and disagreeable in taste. Unfortunately the addition of flavouring agents and mask the unpleasant taste is contraindicated.

c) The solution occasionally causes a reversible tissue irritation manifested by gingival blanching. The reaction usually occurs in individuals with poor gingival health.

d) Pigmentation of teeth after application occurs. The pigmentation ahs a characteristic light brown colour, it usually appears in association with carious lesions and hypocalicified regions of the teeth and around margins of restorations[16].

Figure 4: Comparison of topical fluoride agents[4]

	Characteristics	NaF	SnF_2	APF
1.	Percentage	2%	8%	1.23%
2.	ppm fluoride	9200	19,500	12,300
3.	Frequency of application	4 at weekly interval at ages 3, 7, 11 and 13	1 or 2 / years	1 or 2 / years
4.	Taste	Bland	Disagreeable	Acidic
5.	Stability	Stable	Unstable	Stable in plastic container
6.	Tooth pigmentation	No	Yes	No
7.	Gingival irritation	No	Occasional Transient	No

FLUORIDE VARNISH

First developed and marketed in the 1960s in the form of sodium fluoride (Duraphat, Colgate, New York, N.Y.) and in the 1970s in the form of silane fluoride (Fluor Protector, Ivoclar Vivadent, Lichtenstein, Germany), fluoride varnishes prolong contact between fluoride and enamel. The effectiveness, ease of application and relative safety of these products offer significant advantages over other topical fluoride treatments, such as gels and rinses[44]. In North America, sodium fluoride varnish was introduced first in Canada, and later in the US when it was cleared by the Food and Drug Administration (FDA) for use as a desensitizing agent and cavity liner. As such, its use for caries prevention in the US is "off-label" (i.e., it is being used for a purpose that has not received FDA approval or clearance). Since its introduction in the United States in the 1990s, its use for the prevention of caries has increased among the dental community[40].

Fluoride varnish is not a consumer product and must be applied by a qualified dental hygienist or dentist. The aim of varnishes is to prolong the contact between fluoride and the tooth enamel and promote the remineralization of damaged enamel[13]. Varnishes are topical and deliver F to the surface and subsurface carious lesions by the formation of deposits of calcium fluoride. The calcium fluoride acts as a F pool and provides F for a prolonged time. F varnishes are indicated for therapeutic applications to control active caries, root surface caries, xerostomia patients, hypersensitive areas of enamel and dentine, and physically or mentally handicapped patients[45].

Fluoride varnish is a concentrated topical fluoride that is applied to the teeth by using a small brush and sets on contact with saliva. The concentration of fluoride varnish is 22600 ppm (2.26%), and the active ingredient is sodium fluoride[16]. As a very small quantity (0.3–0.6 mL containing 6.6–13.2 mg F) is applied by trained professionals the ingested amount is generally considered to be too little to induce any toxic or unwanted effects[46]. The unit dose packaging from most manufacturers provides a specific measured amount (0.25 mg, providing 5 mg of fluoride ion). The application of fluoride varnish during an oral screening is of benefit to children, especially those who may have limited access to dental care. Current American Academy of Pediatric Dentistry recommendations for children at high risk of caries is that fluoride varnish be applied to their teeth every 3 to 6 months[20]. According to the American Dental Association (ADA), two or more applications of fluoride varnish per year are effective in reducing caries prevalence in high risk populations (ADA, 2006). Fluoride varnish is a simple and easy preventive measure that can help avoid costly dental procedures, such as fillings, root canals, crowns, or implants[13]. The 2013 ADA guideline recommends application of fluoride varnish at least every 6 months to both primary and permanent teeth in those subjects at elevated caries risk[16].

Fluoride varnish main components:

The active ingredient of fluoride varnish is usually 5% sodium fluoride. The inactive ingredients in the varnish are essentially there to give some flavooring and to ensure that the fluoride sticks to the tooth surface. Common ingredients include sodium saccharin or xylitol, which is used as a sweetener. Raspberry essence or bubble gum tang can be added into the varnish to give an appealing flavour. Ethanol and beeswax or white wax can be used to form a gel-type structure to stabilize the sodium ions. Shellac and mastic are generally used to provide a flexible, permeable hard surface that prevents the varnish from dissolving rapidly in saliva. Kolophonium or colophony is often added into the varnish as a flow enhancer[47].

Mode of action of fluoride varnish

Although a complete understanding of the mechanism of fluoride action in dental caries is still being investigated, it has been found that the application of concentrated fluoride ions in fluoride varnish forms globules of calcium fluoride-like material on the tooth surface[48]. These globules are stabilized by protein phosphate in the mouth. They are fairly insoluble and act as an insoluble reservoir of fluoride at neutral pH. When there is a cariogenic challenge, the pH is lowered and the dissolution rate of these globules increases. Fluoride is thus released and this increases the saturation of calcium and phosphate ions in plaque fluid by lowering the solubility constant of calcium and phosphate ions. This helps to prevent the dissolution of calcium and phosphate from the tooth mineral and/or increases the rate of remineralization or reprecipitation of the lost minerals. This mechanism can explain how the topical application of a fluoride varnish, two to three times a year, can result in long-term caries reduction. The action of fluoride in fluoride varnish makes it useful in caries prevention and caries arrest. Moreover, fluoride varnish is also used to treat dentinal hypersensitivity. Again, although a complete understanding of the mechanism of dentinal hypersensitivity is still being sought, many researchers have accepted the hydrodynamic theory. This theory explains how the occlusion caused by a layer of fluoride varnish, covering the open dentinal tubules, helps to decrease sensitivity. Laboratory study findings show that fluoride uptake can be enhanced by laser, and hence an improved results for treating hypersensitive teeth[49].

Furthermore, the globules of calcium fluoride-like material may act as reservoirs to push the released fluoride into the dentinal tubules, possibly remineralizing internally and blocking the flow of dentinal fluid. This dual mechanism of covering the tubules and in situ remineralization provides relief against tooth sensitivity. In the United States, Duraphat varnish was cleared by the FDA as an anti-hypersensitivity agent in 1994[47].

Instructions for Use

Fluoride varnish must be applied by a dentist, dental auxiliary professional, physician, nurse, or other health care professional, depending on the practice regulations in each state. It should not be dispensed to families to apply at home. Application of fluoride varnish is most commonly performed at the time of a well-child visit[16]. The application of varnish is not intended to adhere permanently to a tooth, but should remain in contact with the surface for several hours. Tooth brushing or wiping or drying with cotton rolls or gauze is adequate to clean the teeth before varnish application. The varnish is then applied with a microapplicator, or a fine brush, to surfaces of the teeth where caries is most likely to initiate. Even with slight moisture in the oral cavity, the varnish will quickly set on contact with teeth. Afterwards, patients are advised to avoid brushing or flossing until the next day. For the first four hours after applications, patients are recommended to only drink water and eat soft foods (Azarpazhooh, 2008)[13]. The following day, they should resume brushing twice daily with fluoridated toothpaste[16].

Advantages:

a) Well tolerated by infants and young children

b) Has a prolonged therapeutic effect

c) Can be applied by both dental and nondental health professionals in a variety of settings[16].

d) The application method is simple and quick

e) Requiring no special equipment[18]

f) Small volume, less time

g) Well received by patients (less discomfort)

h) Less likely to be swallowed in comparison to other forms[36]

i) Slow release of fluoride over time[13].

j) It is suitable for the special needs populations such as very young children, autistic persons and patients with management problems, such as the mentally or physically handicapped.

k) The simplicity of its application makes it very suitable and useful in outreach dental services[47].

Disadvantage:

a) Poor aesthetic effect because a yellow film of varnish remains on the teeth for several hours after application and this needs to be removed by brushing.

b) There is also a temporary discoloration of teeth after varnish application.

c) Fluoride varnishes may have an effect on colour stability of aesthetic restorative materials.

d) Some patients dislike its presence as a thin film on their teeth

e) Taste of the varnish objectionable[47].

Fluoride varnish products:

Figure 5: Common fluoride varnishes and their manufacturers[47]

Product	Manufacturer
Duraphat	Colgate-Palmolive, Canton, MA, USA
Fluor Protector	Ivoclar/Vivadent, Amherst, NY, USA
Duraflor	Pharma Science, Montreal, Canada
CavityShield	OMNII Oral Pharmaceuticals, West Palm Beach, FL, USA
Bifluorid 12	Voco, Germany
Mirafluorid	Hager and Werken, Germany
Carex	Voss, Norway (no longer available)

Duraphat was the first commercially available fluoride varnish. Other common fluoride varnishes include Fluor Protector, Duraflor, CavityShield, Bifluorid 12, Mirafluorid. and Carex (developed in Norway but is no longer available in the market). Experimental fluoride varnishes reported in literature include CDB, an experimental NaF-ethanol varnish which fosters a high fluoride uptake in enamel, and a white fluoride varnish which was found to have good patient acceptance[50]. Duraphat is a 5% NaF preparation. It has been widely used in European countries since the 1980s and is also widely used in the Middle East, Australia, New Zealand, and many countries in Asia. Since 1997, Duraphat in tubes containing 10 mL of varnish has been distributed by Colgate Oral Pharmaceuticals in the United States after obtaining approval for use in dentistry there by the Food and Drug Administration (FDA). There are a number of clinical studies on Duraphat, many of which found it effective in caries prevention in children. At present, it is the most commonly used fluoride varnish and is used in more than 40 countries throughout the world[47].

Fluor Protector is a difluorosaline agent introduced in the mid-1970s; some claimed that Fluor Protector could result in a high fluoride uptake by enamel. Fluor Protector contains 0.7% fluoride in a polyurethane varnish and, unlike Duraphat, has acidic properties. It is available in 1.0 mL ampules and 0.4 mL single-unit doses. In the USA, it is used in a 0.1% fluoride concentration and is marketed as a cavity varnish to seal and prevent the permeation of fluids and metal ions[47].

Duraflor is a 5% NaF varnish that is available in 10 mL tubes. It includes xylitol (a sweetener) and bubblegum flavouring to increase patient acceptance. Reports have suggested it could prevent caries development and also could arrest caries progression[51].

CavityShield contains 5% NaF in a neutral resin and is packaged in single-use doses of 0.25 mL and 0.4 mL with an uniform fluoride content. An advertised advantage of CavityShield is that the unit dose can be mixed easily and applied to teeth, eliminating the concern of administering an unknown dose of fluoride[47].

Bifluorid 12 contains both NaF (2.7% F-) and CaF2 (2.9% F-). A study reported that this NaF/CaF2 varnish deposited more fluoride on the surface of demineralized enamel than NaF varnish alone[52].

Mirafluorid is a fluoride varnish based on an emulsion. It contains an aqueous polymer layer which allows fluoride to diffuse and is dissolved in saliva. It is free of solvents and can be applied under moist conditions. Mirafluorid is available in bottles containing 5 mL of varnish with 0.15 % NaF. This concentration of fluoride is low compared with other common varnishes. The manufacturer claims that it has equal efficacy with other fluoride varnishes in caries prevention. However, a study found it deposited less structurally bound fluoride on both demineralized and sound enamel than 5% NaF varnish[53].

FLUORIDATED PROPHYLACTIC PASTE

Prophylatic pasts with fluoride were developed to allow the practitioner the opportunity to provide both the cleaning and the fluoride application one step. The use of fluoride prophylaxis paste containing 1% NaF in a small group of children can be traced back to Bibby (1946). They reported caries reductions from 25% to 43% depend on the number of treatments. In the beginning these pastes contained NaF or SnF_2 with pumice or silex as abrasive and were never marketed. 1st marked prophylaxis paste contained SnF_2 as active ingredient and Zirconium silicate as the abrasive[54].

It has been mentioned that surface enamel contains higher levels of fluoride than is found in internal layers, therefore, a prophylaxis removes a fluoride rich layer. If prophylaxis pastes containing fluoride are used, the lost fluoride is replenished and there is small but significant, net gain in the concentration of fluoride (Stearns – 1973)[22].

PROFESSIONALLY FLUORIDE FOAMS

Fluoride gels and foams are generally administered by a dentist for patients who are at high risk for dental caries. For individuals at a moderate risk for caries, fluoride gels or foams are recommended every 6 months (Marinho, 2002). High risk individuals can receive gel treatments as often as every 3 months (Marinho, 2002). Some gels and foams can be self-applied at home with the aid of a toothbrush, but the concentration of fluoride in these products is significantly lower. In a professional setting, a dentist will load the gel or foam into a tray then insert it into the patient's mouth. Approximately 5 ml of gel is used in a single tray (Marinho, 2002). The patient bites down on the tray for about four minutes. Afterwards, patients are advised not to rinse, eat, or drink for about 30 minutes in order to prolong contact between the fluoride and tooth enamel. A dentist can also make a tray that is custom fitted for a patient's teeth, and fluoride treatments can be loaded into this tray and be used overnight at home. Fluoride gels do contain abrasives, such as calcium carbonate, dehydrated silica gels, hydrated aluminum oxides, magnesium carbonate, phosphate salts and silicates, which can be found in toothpaste (Marinho, 2002). The concentration of fluoride in gels is significantly higher than that which is found in toothpaste. Fluoride gels can include sodium fluoride, stannous fluoride and acidulated phosphate fluoride. Typically, gels will consist of 12,300 ppm F (Marinho, 2002). Because this is such a highly concentrated form of fluoride, excessive ingestion of gels can lead to acute toxicity. Nausea, vomiting, headache and abdominal pain are symptoms if overexposure of fluoride occurs (Marinho, 2002). Because of the risk of over ingestion the use of gels in young children is not recommended (Marinho, 2002)[55].

METHODS OF APPLICATION OF TOPICAL FLUORIDE

The two most common operator applied topical fluoride methods are the :

1. Paint on technique
2. The tray technique.

While a spray application has been tried (Depaola – 1967) it was never generally recommended. There is a controversy regarding cleaning of teeth prior to a professional topical fluoride application.

Mc Nee et al (1980) have shown that NaF diffuses rapidly through plaque, which is in agreement with the observations of Toyston-Bechal et al 1976 that plaque is no barrier to fluoride deposition in enamel from topical solutions. Also it is in plaque removal prior to topical fluoride application may not alter the clinical effectiveness of the application, it is prudent at this stage to conclude that the harmful effect of plaque as a major cause of caries and gingivitis for out weighs its beneficial effect as a vehicle in which fluoride may act and that it should be removed.

a. **Paint-On Technique-** The patient is instructed to rinse the mouth, the teeth are isolated using cotton rolls. Saliva absorbers may also be used to cover the parotid duct openings and a saliva ejector should be placed beneath the tongue for maximum saliva control. Either a half mouth (left or rt. quadrants) or quadrant is isolated and treated. The isolated teeth are dried with compressed air Hattah et al has reported that one minute air drying will result in significantly more fluoride uptake by the outer enamel. The application is performed by merely swabbing or painting the various tooth surfaces with the cotton applicator thoroughly moistened with fluoride solution the swabbing procedure is performed methodically by repeated loading of the cotton application with one fluoride solution.

Precautions

a) Use of only required amount of gel / solution.

b) Positioning the patient in an upright position.

c) Using efficient saliva aspiration or suctioning apparatus.

d) Patient should be allowed to thoroughly expectorate upon completion of the fluoride application.

e) The strict following of above said procedures will reduce the swallowing of 10-30 mg of F to 2 mg by young children which might lead to dental fluorosis.

b. **Tray-Technique-** Armamentarium consists simply of a suitable tray and the fluoride gel. Different types of tray made out of polyvinyl, wax, paper or foam are available. The tray selected should include the whole of patient arch with enough depth to reach beyond the neck of the teeth and contract the alveolar mucosa to prevent saliva from diluting mucosa. At present, disposable soft Styrofoam trays are available which can be bent to insert in mouth, which are more comfortable and both arches can be treated simultaneously. In some earlier trays a soft sponge like material was used which squeezed the gel against the teeth when the patient was asked to bite lightly to ensure the flow of material interproximally[12].

DIFFERENT TECHNIQUE OF FLUORIDE APPLICATION

1. The Knutson's technique- Initially cleaning and polishing of the teeth is done in only the1st of the four application . an upper and opposing lower quadrant are opposing lower quadrants are isolated with cotton rolls and the teeth are dried thoroughly. 2%NaF is then applied with cotton applicators and is permitted to dry on the teeth for about 4 minutes. The procedure is repeated for the remaining quadrants. After completion of the treatment the patient is instructed to avoid eating, drinking or rinsing for 30 min so as to prolong the availability of fluoride ion to react with the tooth surfaces. $2^{nd}, 3^{rd}, 4^{th}$ application are given at weekly intervals. A full series of four treatments is recommended at ages 3,7,11 and 13.

2. Muller's technique - The teeth are then isolated with cotton roll and dried preferably with compressed air . Either a quadrant or half of the mouth can be treated at one time. Quadrant to be treated should be kept free of saliva and if possible a saliva ejector should be used. A freshly prepared solution of stannous fluoride is applied continuously to the teeth with cotton applicator so that the teeth are kept moist with the solution for 4 min and a replication of solution to a particular tooth is done every 15-30 sec . The recommended frequency of application is one per year[30].

3. Mercer and Muller technique – same as Muller's except that the teeth are kept moist for 30 secs instead of 4 min.

4. Dubbing and Muller technique - This is a combination of a 4 min topical application of fluoride solution preceded by a prophylaxis with a stannous fluoride paste, each surface of each tooth being treated for 10 secs. Unwaxed silk floss is used interproximally. Szwejda modified this technique by applying the solution for 30 seconds instead of for 4 mins[18].

5. The Englader technique- In this method TF is applied in specific maxillary and mandibular mouth pieces made from sheets of thermoplastic vinyl resin. Applications are made for 3 minutes.

6. Szwejda – Knutson multiple – chair technique- Essentially the same as the Knutson method but the time taken / child is greatly reduced by using several chairs[47].

RECOMMENDATION IN USE OF PROFESSIONALLY APPLIED TOPICAL FLUORIDES

ADA Council on Scientific Affairs recommendations for the use of professionally applied topical fluoride. The Council does point out that laboratory data has demonstrated the equivalence of fluoride release of topical fluoride foam to topically-applied gels. However, only two clinical trials have been published that have evaluated the fluoride foam's effectiveness. Due to the scarcity of clinical information, the recommendations of fluoride varnish and gels have not been extrapolated to fluoride foams. Furthermore, since there is insufficient evidence that addresses the efficacy of sodium fluoride (NaF) versus acidulated phosphate fluoride (APF), the recommendations do not distinguish between these two formulations. Fluoride gel and foam application times should not be less than four minutes. Although evidence suggests that fluoride varnish is effective in caries prevention, the Council does recognize that its recommendation for fluoride varnish remains an "off-label" use of this product, as fluoride varnishes have only been approved by the US Food and Drug Administration (FDA) for the treatment of hypersensitive exposed root surfaces and also as a cavity varnish. Furthermore, it is recommended that all age and risk groups use the appropriate amount of fluoride-containing toothpaste when brushing twice a day and additional preventive interventions (e.g., at home fluoride products, pit and fissure sealants, anti-bacterial therapy) should be considered for individuals in the moderate and high risk caries groups[56].

Figure 6: Evidence Based Clinical Recommendations for Professionally Applied Topical Fluoride[36].

Risk Category	< 6 Years	6 to 18 Years	> 18 Years
Low	May not receive additional benefit from professional topical fluoride application	May not receive additional benefit from professional topical fluoride application	May not receive additional benefit from professional topical fluoride application
Moderate	Varnish application at 6-month intervals	Varnish application at 6-month intervals OR Fluoride gel applications at 6-month intervals	Varnish application at 6-month intervals OR Fluoride gel applications at 6-month intervals
High	Varnish application at 6-month intervals OR Varnish application at 3-month intervals	Varnish application at 6-month intervals or Varnish application at 3-month intervals or Fluoride gel application at 6-month intervals or Fluoride gel application at 3-month intervals	Varnish application at 6-month intervals or Varnish application at 3-month intervals or Fluoride gel application at 6-month intervals or Fluoride gel application at 3-month intervals

Figure 7: Summary of the Recommendations for the Use of Fluoride Regimens in Contemporary Pediatric Dental Practice[30]

Fluoride regimen	Recommendations
Dietary supplements	• Assay patient's primary source of drinking water; consider other sources of fluoride intake • Consider delaying supplementation until after eruption of permanent first molars • Ensure that parents understand risks/benefits of supplementation • Instruct patient to chew/swish supplement prior to swallowing • Prescribe no more than 120 mg F • No benefit to prenatal administration
Dentifrices	• Use in children <2 yrs old should be based on caries risk assessment • Tooth-brushing for young child should be done by adult; brushing by older child should be supervised by adult • Use pea-sized dab of dentifrice in children with immature swallowing reflexes; older children can use larger amounts • Brush with fluoride toothpaste twice daily
Mouthrinses	• Reserve for use in children with moderate/high caries risk • Reserve for use in children who have mastered swallowing reflex • Recommend alcohol-free preparations

Self-applied gels/pastes (5000 ppm F)	• Reserve for patients in fluoride-deficient communities who are at increased risk for caries • Application should be done by adult for young child, and supervised by adult for older child • Application period should be 4 minutes • Allow patient to expectorate freely after application; postpone eating/drinking for 30 minutes • Use with caution in children who have not mastered swallowing reflex • Monitor effectiveness; terminate regimen when feasible
Professionally applied gel/foam (12,300 ppm F)	• Application frequency based on caries risk assessment • Follow a pumice prophylaxis with fluoride application • Use minimum amount of gel/foam necessary to cover teeth • Seat patient upright, use suction to reduce swallowing of product • Apply for 4 minutes • Allow patient to expectorate freely after application; postpone eating/drinking for 30 minutes
Fluoride varnish (22,600 ppm F)	• Use after pumice prophylaxis as noted for gel/foam application • Use in alternative restorative technique to arrest lesions in young, precooperative patients • Have patient refrain from eating/drinking for 30 minutes after application • Have patient postpone brushing teeth until following morning

RECENT ADVANCE IN TOPICAL FLUORIDES

New /or improved fluoride products are entering the marketplace at an increased rate; these products include toothpastes, fluoride varnishes, fluoride containing whitening agents, and other fluoride containing cleaning products.

In early 2011, after years of review and evaluation, the Centers for Disease Control and Prevention (CDC), Environmental Protection Agency (EPA), and the American Dental Association (ADA). CDC, EPA, and the ADA proposed a modification to their recommendations for the amount of fluoride in drinking water to be 0.7 µg/ml (ppm) at all places in the United States. Thus, until 2011, the CDC and the ADA had recommended that the amount of fluoride in drinking water should range from 0.7 ppm in warmer climates to 1.2 ppm in cooler climates.

There are some recent studies in which the amount of fluoride made available in the oral cavity during tooth brushing (for approximately 2 min) was measured. It seems that in developing regions of the world, there are toothpastes marketed that contain the total fluoride as indicated on the label, but they do not release sufficient fluoride during use to prevent caries. This is due to the composition of the toothpaste which can render a significant amount of the fluoride unavailable[57].

In 2005, a stannous fluoride sodium hexametaphosphate (SFSH) formula was introduced offering protection against a broad range of health and cosmetic conditions commonly experienced by patients. Sodium hexametaphosphate was first introduced in a dentifrice in 2000. It provides better coverage and retention on the tooth surface, thus increasing its ability to inhibit both calculus and stain formation on the enamel surface[58].

Fluoride releasing dental restorative materials may provide an additional benefit in preventive dentistry. Comparison of fluoride ion release was made from four different dental restorations (Fuji Vll, Fuji II LC, Dyract, and Z350) in deionized water from day 1 until day 5. The result showed significantly different fluoride ion release from all of them. The fluoride release was highest in Fuji VII, followed by Fuji II LC, Dyract, and Z350. The result also revealed a significant association of fluoride ion release from dental restorations in deionized water and artificial saliva, except for Z350 (P = 0.787). There was greater amount of fluoride release by all the tested materials in deionized water compared with artificial saliva[59].

A new system has been introduced in dentistry for achieving a constant rate of continuous fluoride release for a longer period in the oral cavity which is the intraoral fluoride releasing device to be used in highrisk groups (Mirth et al., 1982; Kula et al., 1987; Toumba and Curzon, 2005)[60].

Thus, fluoride in various forms, i.e., varnishes, rinses, foams, gels, dentifrices, slow releasing devices, prophylaxis paste, remineralizing agents, and in restorative materials, is now available to dental professionals for use in clinical practice and to be used by patients at home[61].

DISCUSSION

The WHO Oral Health Programme continues to emphasize the importance of public health approaches to the effective use of fluorides for the prevention of dental caries in the 21st century. Everyone should be encouraged to brush daily with a fluoride toothpaste. In addition, where the incidence and prevalence of dental caries in the community is high to moderate, or where there are firm indications that the incidence of caries is increasing, an additional source of fluoride should be considered. It should be emphasized that "topical" fluorides such as toothpaste can also have a "systemic" effect when they are inadvertently ingested by young children. Indeed, three independent studies in Australia, Canada and the USA indicate that 47–72% of dental fluorosis in children can be attributed to the systemic effect of fluoride toothpastes . Dispensing a pea-sized amount of toothpaste, encouraging parents to supervise toothbrushing by their young children, and the use of toothpastes containing less fluoride by young children are approaches to ameliorating this problem. It is recommended that dental fluorosis be monitored periodically to detect increases in or higher-than-acceptable levels of fluorosis[30,37,110].

Findings from extensive clinical trials on the efficacy of fluoride dentifrices and/or other self-applied fluoride agents, as well as on professionally applied fluoride treatments, are relevant to strategies to arrest initial lesions and the most effective interventions in treating high-caries-risk persons. Not all fluoride agents and treatments are equal. Different fluoride compounds, different vehicles, and vastly different concentrations of fluoride have been used with different frequency and duration of application . All of these variables influence the clinical outcome with respect to caries prevention. The efficacy of topical fluoride depends on a) the concentration of fluoride used, b) the frequency with which it is applied and the duration of application, and c) the specific fluoride compound used[62,63].

Regarding the concentration of fluoride used, most fluoride dentifrice studies have shown a dose/response effect, and the trends in clinical effectiveness of professionally applied topical fluoride agents are similar. With respect to the frequency of topical fluoride application, in studies using the same commercial stannous fluoride dentifrice, the efficacy of unsupervised once-per-day or adlibitum use was about a 21 percent caries reduction, whereas the efficacy of supervised thrice-per-day use was about a 45 percent caries reduction.Marthaler found that in studies using fluoride brush-on gels or solutions, those that employed fifteen or more applications per year had 40 to 50 percent caries reductions, whereas those with four to five applications per year were less efficacious.

In vitro testing of both NaF and APF solutions has shown that fluoride uptake is time related, and in the case of APF solutions the most rapid uptake occurs during the first four minutes. Although some manufacturers claim that their brand of gel or foam will provide near maximum uptake in one minute, these products lack testing for clinical efficacy. Therefore, the recommended duration of application of APF agents should be four minutes. Fluoride varnishes adhere to tooth surfaces, permitting prolonged fluoride exposure and uptake. Nevertheless, there is a consistency of results in that the more concentrated the fluoride and the greater the frequency of application, the greater the caries reduction. The fact that topical treatments differ in efficacy is often ignored by some who think all such treatments are equivalent. Other factors besides efficacy, such as safety, practicality, cost and compliance, influence the clinician's choice of preventive therapy[63].

The preventive effect of fluoride varnish on primary teeth varies according to age and risk of dental caries. Fluoride varnish releases fluoride during the cariogenic challenge and spreads through the enamel, reducing the progression of carious lesions. Although some authors are in agreement in relation to its effectiveness in reducing the incidence of dental caries in primary teeth of children six years old or less, the evidence of its inhibitory effect on this dentition is limited and evidence on its effectiveness is still insufficient[101].

Fluoride has its greatest effect as a topically applied agent. Topical fluoride applications of gels and solutions have been shown in clinical trials to greatly reduce dental caries. However, much of the fluoride was lost in the first 24 h as it leached away. It was found that a longer exposure time to the enamel increased the efficiency of the topical fluoride and produced fluorapatite that is more acid resistant than hydroxyapatite with its naturally occurring carbonate inclusions. Fluoride varnish is a toxicologically safe way of exposing the enamel to fluoride for longer periods of time than gels or solutions, and it results in a deeper penetration of the fluoride into the enamel surface Clinical trials have shown a significant reduction in dental caries with the use of fluoride varnish. A study by Arends and Schuthof showed that a 24-h exposure of enamel to fluoride after application of fluoride varnishes was sufficient to inhibit demineralization completely as determined by microradiography and micro-hardness tests[65].

The current levels of F in toothpaste do not lead to excessive F exposures in the preschoolers or alternatively, tooth-brushing habits have becomemore appropriate and there is no need for any downward adjustments in the standards for toothpaste. However, the F exposure was widely variable (the 5th percentile and 95th percentile for amount ingested per day being 0.0 and 1451.8 lg), and a mere switch to a toothpaste with different F content or formulation could easily increase the F exposure from this source by several folds. Hence,the ingestion of toothpaste by young children should be constantly monitored with special attention towards flavoured formulations. Because of the highly statistically significant correlations between the fluorides ingested from toothpaste and the amount of toothpaste dispensed , parents should at least assume responsibility for placement of toothpaste and should be reminded to limit the amount of toothpaste used until the child is 6–7 years of age[66].

Toothpaste are the mainstays of fluoride delivery for all. Other modalities should be considered only if the child is at high risk for caries. Care should be exercised in prescribing other modalities of fluoride delivery before age 6, and especially before age 3, because of the risk of dental fluorosis. High-risk groups include children of low socioeconomic status, those whose parents have low levels of education, those who do not regularly attend for dental care and those without dental insurance. High-risk children are those with active caries; those whose siblings have high levels of caries; those with high levels of Streptococcus mutans, cognitive or physical challenges to oral hygiene, or low salivary flow or buffering capacity; and especially those consuming a cariogenic diet and receiving inadequate exposure to fluoride. The most important messages about fluoride recommendations are that making them is more difficult than it used to be and that "more fluoride is not necessarily better"[111].

Fluorosis presence cannot solely be explained by past fluoride intake, our results showed a significant effect on the fluorosis severity score when children reported using larger amount of toothpaste and supplements, which points to the value of using fluorosis as a biomarker for past fluoride exposure. Numerous previous studies have shown significant associations between these factors and increased fluorosis risk[78].

Fluoride mouth-rinsing is very effective for preventing dental caries, is both safe and easy to apply and is a public health method based on scientific evidence. For these reasons, it is estimated that fluoride mouth-rinsing is being performed in groups and at home by about

100 million people throughout the world. Fluoride mouth-rinsing is thus an important means for preventing caries in permanent teeth in almost all life stages[96].

The fluoride content and its release from restorative materials should be high without altering its physical properties and undue degradation of the filling. An initial high level of fluoride release in the vicinity of restoration will reduce the viability of bacteria thus inhibit dental caries by inducing remineralization of enamel/dentin[102].

The mode of action of fluoride has an essential role in the further development of products and programmes for caries prevention. In the past, the cariostatic effect of fluoride was attributed to the incorporation of fluoride in the hydroxyapatite crystal lattice and the reduced solubility of the so-formed fluoridated hydroxyapatite[1,2].

CONCLUSIONS

The primary caries-preventive effects of fluoride result from its topical contact with enamel and through its antibacterial actions. Therefore, therapeutic use of fluoride for children should focus on regimens that maximize topical contact, preferably in lower-dose, higher-frequency approaches. Clinicians should be aware that the level of evidence for most fluoride regimens is fair at best. Until stronger evidence is available, current best practice includes recommending twice-daily use of a dentifrice containing 1,000 ppm F for children in optimally fluoridated and fluoride-deficient communities, coupled with professional application of topical fluoride gel, foam, or varnish. The addition of other fluoride regimens—supplements, mouthrinses, and self-applied gels—should be based on periodic caries risk assessments. Clinicians should keep in mind that the additive effects of multiple fluoride modalities exhibit diminishing returns. Fluoride products should be used in proven, approved regimens, and steps should be taken to reduce the unnecessary ingestion of fluoride by young children.

Fluoride given the importance of preventive care in reducing childhood diseases, it is a public health concern that caregivers' refusal of immunizations is significantly related to their refusal of topical fluoride. This has implications for pediatric medicine and dentistry in terms of increased childhood disease rates, reduced benefits associated with herd immunity, and potential widening of health disparities. Future research should identify the common social and behavioral factors related to caregivers' refusal of various types of preventive care with the goal of developing multidisciplinary strategies to help caregivers make optimal preventive care decisions for children.

The role of F in oral health has been studied for many decades and evidence found to support topical, but not systemic, F as being beneficial. However, it must be emphasized that tooth decay (dental caries) is not caused by F deficiency. Hence F supplementation will never reverse active or gross carious lesions. Therefore, in order to reduce dental decay in populations with a high caries risk, other measures, such as patient counselling and guidance about oral hygiene and food selection, must be taken in conjunction with the F delivery .

Fluoride continues to be the cornerstone of dental caries prevention throughout the world, and there are a variety of sources of fluoride that may contribute to the dietary intake of fluoride. Even though Mexico City is considered a non-endemic area for dental fluorosis according to its low concentration of fluoride in drinking water, the children in our study presented epidemiological indicators of overexposure to fluoride. Our data revealed a urinary excretion within the normal limits established and reported by other authors, but epidemiological indexes showed simultaneously high prevalences of caries and dental fluorosis. Because our knowledge is incomplete regarding the amount, duration, and timing of fluoride ingestion that can result in dental fluorosis, however, further research is clearly needed before definitive recommendations can be made regarding the use of fluorides, including the recommended dietary intake of fluoride. Further longitudinal studies are needed to determine the safe fluorine dose for Mexican children, taking in account age, nutritional status, altitude, geographical location and weather, among other factors.

Carious tooth destruction results from episodes of demineralization of tooth structure exceeding remineralization over time. Consequently, to optimize the possibility for recurrent caries inhibition, a sustained level of fluoride release over time from a restorative material-adhesive system is necessary. Since the intrinsic fluoride release from fluoridated restorative materials and adhesives declines with time, the capacity for a restoration to exhibit anticarious activity will be determined by the material's ability to demonstrate fluoride recharge also.

For children who have been using fluoride toothpaste for many years and have little or no caries, the evidence is less clear. In the short term, little benefit is likely from topical fluorides and even a possible longer-term effect can be expected to be of minor value from the clinical point of view. For low risk individuals who received systemic fluorides during the period of tooth formation and who are using fluoride toothpaste, little or no advantage from topical fluoride will be produced Should the individual change his lifestyle and move from the low risk to the high risk category and early lesions be identified, then topical fluorides will be of benefit.

Dental caries is an infectious disease yet the application of this concept in practice is limited.

Accordingly, antimicrobial approaches, directed at both mothers and at young children, have an important place in tooth decay prevention and control. Antiseptics, chlorhexidine varnish and PVP-iodine, as well as xylitol chewing gum used by mothers, have been shown to be effective in inhibiting carious lesion incidence, but definitive trials are needed.

Fluorides remain the most effective agents but are not widely disseminated to the neediest.

Fluoride varnish provides a relatively effective topical preventive for very young children, yet definitive trials of its application in primary care practice have not been conducted. Scientific advances outside the U.S. have suggested the potential of silver diammine fluoride, but it is not FDA approved and no research has been carried out in the U.S. Data support effectiveness and safety of xylitol, but adoption is not widespread and additional research is needed on formulations and vehicles to increase access. Dental sealants are of unquestioned benefit and remain a mainstay of public policy yet, after decades of research, widespread use has not occurred. Definitive trials are needed of new materials that can be used on erupting teeth.

BIBLIOGRAPHY

1. Stooky GK, Jackson RD, Ferreira G, Analoui M. Dental caries diagnosis. Dent Clin of North Amer.1999; 43(4):665-677.

2. Karlinsey R.L.,Pfarrer A.M. Fluoride Plus Functionalized β-TCP:A Promising Combination for Robust Remineralization. Adv Dent Res.2012;24(2):48-52.

3. Murray JJ, Rugg-Gunn AJ, Jenkins GN. Fluorides in caries prevention. 3rd ed. Oxford: Butterworth-Heinemann Ltd, 1991. Ten Cate J. Current concepts on the theories of the mechanism of action of fluoride. Acta Odontol Scand.1999;57:325-329

4. Newbrun E Topical Fluorides in Caries Prevention and Management: A North American Perspective. J Dent Edu.2001;65(10):1078- 1083.

5. Olympio K P K et al. Urinary fluoride output in children following the use of a dual-fluoride varnish formulation. J Appl Oral Sci.2009; 17(3):179-183.

6. Irish Oral Health Services Guideline Initiative. Topical Fluorides Evidence-based guidance on the use of topical fluorides for caries prevention in children and adolescents in Ireland. 2008.

7. Buzalaf MA, Pessan JP, Honório HM, ten Cate JM. Mechanisms of action of fluoride for caries control. Monogr Oral Sci. 2011; 22: 97-114.

8. Fincham AG, Moradian-Oldak J, Simmer JP. The structural biology of the developing dental enamel matrix. J. Struct. Biol.1999; 126: 270-299.

9. Francais en.The use of fluoride in infants and Children. Paediatr Child Health. Canadian Paediatric Society.2002;7(8):569-572.

10. Dean HT. On the epidemiology of fluorine and dental caries. In: Gies WJ (ed). Fluorine in dental public health. New York, NY: New York Institute of Clinical Oral Pathology.1945:19-30.

11. Noda GM. The Controversy over Community Water Fluoridation: An Analysis of its Effects and Reasons Behind the Arguments. University Honors Theses.2016 Available from.http://pdxscholar.library.pdx.edu/honorstheses/2016.[Last accessed on 11 october,2016]

12. Jalili VP, Tewari A. Fluorides and dental caries : A Compendium. 1st ed. Indore: J Indian Dent Assoc ;1986.

13. American Dental Association. Fluoridation Facts. Chicago, IL. Available from http://www.ada.org/sections/professionalResources/pdfs/fluoridation_facts.pdf.[Last accessed on 16 November 2016]

14. Twetman S, Axelsson S, Dahlgren H, Holm AK, Kallestal C, Lagerlof F, Lingstrom P, Mejare I, Nordenram G, Norlund A, Petersson LG, Soder B: Caries-preventive effect of fluoride toothpaste: a systematic review. Acta Odontol Scand.2003; 61:347-355.

15. Ullah R, Zafar M S. Oral and dental delivery of fluoride :A Review. Fluoride J.2015;48(3):195-204.

16. Clark M B, Slayton R L. Fluoride Use in Caries Prevention in the Primary Care Setting. J. Pediatr.2014;134(3):626-633.

17. Kidd EAM. Essentials of dental caries: the disease and its management. 3rd ed. New York: Oxford University Press; 2005.

18. Davies R, Ellwood R, Davies G. The rational use of fluoride toothpaste. Int J Dent Hyg. 2003;1:3-8.

19. Wright JT et al. Fluoride toothpaste efficacy and safety in children younger than six years of age: a systematic review. J Am Dent Assoc. 2014;145(2):182–189.

20. American Academy of Pediatric Dentistry. Guideline on Fluoride Therapy. Chicago, IL:American Academy of Pediatric Dentistry;2013. Available at: www.aapd.org/media/

Policies_Guidelines/G_fluoridetherapy.pdf.Accessed nov 20, 2016.

21. Marinho VC. Evidence based effectiveness of topical fluorides .Adv Dent Res. 2008;20:3-7.

22. Limeback H, Ismail A, Banting D, et al. Canadian Consensus Conference on the appropriate use of fluoride supplements for the prevention of dental caries in children. J Can Dent Assoc.1998;64:636-639.

23. Guidelines on the use of fluoride in children: an EAPD policy document. Eur. Arch. Paediatr. Dent.2009;10 (3):129-135.

24. Carey C M. Focus on Fluorides: Update on the Use of Fluoride for the Prevention of Dental Caries. J Evid Based Dent Pract.2014;14:95-102.

25. Bibby BG. A test of the effect of fluoride-containing dentifrices on dental caries. J Dent Res.1945;24:297-303.

26. Zero D T. Dentifrices, mouthwashes, and remineralization/caries arrestment Strategies. BMC Oral Health 2006;6(1):1-13.

27. Zero DT, Raubertas RF, Fu J, Pedersen AM, Hayes AL, Featherstone JDB: Fluoride concentration in plaque, whole saliva and ductal saliva after application of home-use topical fluorides. J Dent Res.1992;71:1768-1775.

28. Marinho VC, Higgins JP, Sheiham A, Logan S: Fluoride toothpastes for preventing dental caries in children and adolescents.Cochrane Database Syst Rev.2003;1:25-32.

29. Aasenden R, Brudevold F, Richardson B: Clearance of fluoride from the mouth after topical treatment or the use of a fluoride mouthrinse. Arch Oral Biol.1968;13:625-636.

30. Adair S M.Evidence-based Use of Fluoride in Contemporary Pediatric Dental Practice. Pediatr Dent.2006; 28(2):133-142.

31. Tressaud A, Haufe G. Fluorine and health: molecular imaging, biomedical materials and pharmaceuticals.1st ed. Oxford: Elsevier; 2008.

32. Cameron AC, Widmer RP. Handbook of pediatric dentistry. 4th ed. Oxford, UK:Mosby Elsevier; 2013.

33. Driscoll WS, Swango PA, Horowitz AM, Kingman A: Caries-preventive effects of daily and weekly fluoride mouthrinsing in a fluoridated community: final results after 30 months. J Am Dent Assoc.1982;105:1010-1013.

34. Twetman S, Petersson L, Axelsson S, Dahlgren H, Holm AK, Kallestal C, Lagerlof F, Lingstrom P, Mejare I, Nordenram G, Norlund A, Soder B: Caries-preventive effect of sodium fluoride mouthrinses: a systematic review of controlled clinical trials. Acta Odontol Scand.2004;62:223-230.

35. Wei SH, Hattab FN. Enamel fluoride uptake from a new APF foam. Pediatric Dent.1988;10(2):111-114.

36. American Dental Association Council on Scientific Affairs. Professionally applied topical fluoride: evidence-based clinical recommendations. J Am Dent Assoc.2006;137(8):1151-1159.

37. Beltrán-Aguilar ED, Goldstein JW, Lockwood S. Fluoride varnishes: a review of their clinical use, cariostatic mechanism, efficacy and safety. J Am Dent Assoc. 2000;131: 589-596.

38. Ripa LW. Review of the anticaries effectiveness of professionally applied and self-applied topical fluoride gels. J Public Health Dent.1989;49:297-309.

39. Bawden JW. Fluoride varnish: a useful new tool for publichealth dentistry. J Public Health Dent.1998;58:266-269.

40. Autio-Gold J. Fluoride varnishes for everyday practice. Pract Proced Aesthet Dent. 2005;17:398-400.

41. Qgaard B,Seppa L,Rolla G. Professional topical fluoride applications clinical efficacy and mechanism of action.Adv Dent Res.1994;8(2):190-201.

42. Arief EP, Kunarti S. The effect of acidulated phosphate fluoride application on dental enamel surfaces hardness. Dent. J. (Maj. Ked. Gigi)2007;40(3):145-147.

43. Samuel SMW, Rubinstein C. Microhardness of enamel restored with floride and non–flouride raleasing dental materials. Braz Dent J.2001; 12(1):35-38.

44. Azarpazhooh A.Fluoride Varnish in the Prevention of Dental Caries in Children and Adolescents: A Systematic Review. J Can Dent Assoc.2008;74(1):73-79.

45. Davies GM, Bridgman C, Hough D, Davies R. The application of fluoride varnish in the prevention and control of dental caries. Dent Update.2009;36:410-412.

46. Kidd EAM. Essentials of dental caries: the disease and its management. 3rd ed. New York: Oxford University Press; 2005.

47. Chu CH, Lo E. Uses of sodium fluoride varnish in dental practice. Ann Roy Australas Coll Dent Surg.2008;19:58-61.

48. Ogaard B. The cariostatic mechanism of fluoride. Compend Contin Educ Dent.1999;20(1):10-17.

49. Corona SA, Nascimento TN, Catirse AB, Lizarelli RF, Dinelli W, Palma-Dibb RG. Clinical evaluation of low-level laser therapy and fluoride varnish for treating cervical dentinal hypersensitivity. J Oral Rehabil.2003;30:1183-1189.

50. Berg J, Riedy CA, Tercero A. Patient and parental perception of a new fluoride varnish. Compend Contin Educ Dent.2006;27:614-618.

51. Milgrom P, Rothen M, Spadafora A, Skaret E. A case report: arresting dental caries. J Dent Hyg. 2001;75:241-243.

52. Attin T, Hartmann O, Hilgers RD, Hellwig E. Fluoride retention of incipient enamel lesions after treatment with a calcium fluoride varnish in vivo. Arch Oral Biol. 1995;40: 169-174.

53. Attin T, Grieme R, Paque F, Hannig C, Buchalla W, Attin R. Enamel fluoride uptake of a novel water-based fluoride varnish. Arch Oral Biol.2005;50:317-322.

54. Tewari A, Chawla HS, Utreja A. Comparative evaluation of the role of NaF, APF and Duraphat topical fluoride applications in the prevention of dental caries: a 2 1/2 years study. J Indian Soc Pedod Prev Dent.1991; 8(1):28–35.

55. Jiang H, Tai B, Du M, Peng B. Effect of professional application of APF foam on caries reduction in permanent first molars in 6-7-year-old children: 24-month clinical trial. J Dent. 2005; 33(6):469–473.

56. Chu CH, Lo ECM. A review of sodium fluoride varnish. Gen Dent.2006;54:247-253.

57. Carey CM. Focus on Fluorides: Update on the use of Fluoride for the prevention of Dental Caries. JEBDP. 2014;4(2):1–27.

58. Sensabaugh C, Sagel ME. Stannous Fluoride Dentifrice with Sodium Hexametaphosphate. J.D.2009;83:70–78.

59. Nik Noorul Azam bt Nik Yusoff, Ariffin Z, Hassan A, Alam MK. Fluoride Release from Dental Restorations in Deionized Water and Artificial Saliva. IMJ. 2013;20:635–638.

60. Dupare R, Kumar P, Dupare A, Jain R, Chitguppi R. Intraoral Slow Release Fluoride Devices. I J Pre Clin Dent Res. 2014;1:37–41.

61. Bansal A,Ingle NA,Kaur N,Ingle E.Recent advancements in fluoride: A systematic review. J Int Soc Prev Community Dent.2015; 5(5): 341–346.

62. Klein SP.The Cost and Effectiveness of School-based Preventive Dental Care. Am J Public Health.1985;75(4):382-391.

63. Newbrun E.Topical Fluorides in Caries Prevention and Management: A North American Perspective. J Dent Educ. 2001;65(10):1078-1083.

64. Levy SM .An Update on Fluorides and Fluorosis. J Can Dent Assoc.2003; 69(5): 286–291.

65. Eakle WS, Featherstone JDB, Weintraub JA, Shain SG, Gansky SA. Salivary fluoride levels following application of fluoride varnish or fluoride rinse. Community Dent Oral Epidemiol.2004; 32: 462–469.

66. Tan BS, Razak IA. Fluoride exposure from ingested toothpaste in 4–5-year-old Malaysian children. Community Dent Oral Epidemiol.2005; 33: 317–325.

67. Zero DT.Dentifrices, mouthwashes, and remineralization/caries arrestment strategies BMC Oral Health.2006;6(1):1-13.

68. Arnold WH. Effect of fluoride toothpastes on enamel demineralization.BMC Oral Health. 2006;6(8):1-6.

69. Hong L, Levy SM, Broffitt B, Warren JJ, Kanellis MJ, Wefel JS, Dawson DV. Timing of fluoride intake in relation to development of fluorosis on maxillary central incisors. Community Dent Oral Epidemiol.2006; 34: 299–309.

70. Weintraub JA, Ramos-Gomez F, Jue B, Shain V. Fluoride Varnish Efficacy in Preventing Early Childhood Caries. J Dent Res. 2006; 85(2): 172–176.

71. Arief E ,Kunarti S.The effect of acidulated phosphate fluoride application on dental enamel surfaces hardness. Dent. J. (Maj. Ked. Gigi).2007; 40(3):145-147.

72. Aminabadi NA, Balaei E, Pouralibaba F. The Effect of 0.2% Sodium Fluoride Mouthwash in Prevention of Dental Caries According to the DMFT Index.. J. dent. res. dent. clin. dent. prospect.2007;1(2):71-76.

73. Goldman AS, Yee R, Holmgren CJ , Benzian H. Global affordability of fluoride toothpaste. Global Health.2008;4(7):4-8.

74. Vogel G.L., Chow L.C. ,Carey C.M. Calcium Pre-Rinse Greatly Increases Overnight Salivary Fluoride after a 228 ppm Fluoride Rinse. Caries Res.2008;42:401–404.

75. Deepti A, Jeevarathan J, Muthu MS, Rathna PV, Chamundeswari. Effect of Fluoride Varnish on Streptococcus mutans Count in Saliva of Caries Free Children Using Dentocult SM Strip Mutans Test: A Randomized Controlled Triple Blind Study. Int J Clin Pediatr Dent .2008;1(1):1-9.

76. Prabhakar AR , Arali V. Comparison of the Remineralizing Effects of Sodium Fluoride and Bioactive Glass Using Bioerodible Gel Systems. J Dent Res Dent Clin Dent Prospect 2009; 3(4):117-121.

77. Naumova EA, Gaengler P, Zimmer S , Arnold WH. Influence of Individual Saliva Secretion on Fluoride Bioavailability. Open Dent J. 2010; 4:185-190.

78. Martinez-Mier EA, Soto-Rojas AE. Differences in exposure and biological markers of fluoride among White and African American children. J Public Health Dent.2010:1-7.

79. .Botta AC, Mollica FB,Ribeiro CF, Araujo MAM, Nicoló RD,Balducci I.Influence of topical acidulated phosphate fluoride on surface roughness of human enamel and different restorative materials. Rev. odonto cienc. 2010;25(1):83-87.

80. Song W, Toda S,Komiyama E,Komiyama K,Arakawa Y,He D, Arakawa H. Fluoride Retention following the Professional Topical Application of 2% Neutral Sodium Fluoride Foam.Inter J Dent.2011:1-6.

81. Tut OK, Milgrom PM. Topical Iodine And Fluoride Varnish Combined Is More Effective Than Fluoride Varnish Alone For Protecting Erupting First Permanent Molars: A Retrospective Cohort Study. J Public Health Dent. 2010 ; 70(3): 249–252.

82. Jimenez-Farfan MD, Hernandez-Guerrero JC, Juarez-Lopez LA, Jacinto-Aleman LF, Fuente-Hernandez JD.Fluoride Consumption and Its Impact on Oral Health.Int. J. Environ. Res. Public Health. 2011;8:148-160.

83. Oganessian E , Ivancakova R , Lencova E, Broukal Z. Alimentary fluoride intake in preschool children. BMC Public Health .2011;11:1-6.

84. Erdem AP, Sepet E, Kulekci G, Trosola SC, Guven Y.Effects of Two Fluoride Varnishes and One Fluoride/Chlorhexidine Varnish on Streptococcus mutans and Streptococcus sobrinus Biofilm Formation in Vitro. Int. J. Med. Sci. 2012; 9(2):129-136.

85. Peros K, Mestrovic K, Anic-Milosevic S, Rosin-Grget K, Slaj M. Antimicrobial effect of different brushing frequencies with fluoride toothpaste on Streptococcus mutans and Lactobacillus species in children with fixed orthodontic appliances. Korean J Orthod. 2012;42(5):263-269.

86. Erdem AP, Sepet E, Kulekci G,Trosola SC, Guven Y.Effects of Two Fluoride Varnishes and One Fluoride/Chlorhexidine Varnish on Streptococcus mutans and Streptococcus sobrinus Biofilm Formation in Vitro Int. J. Med. Sci. 2012;9(2):129-136.

87. Naumova E A, Kuehnl P, Hertenstein P , Markovic L, Jordan R A, Gaengler P , Arnold WH. Fluoride bioavailability in saliva and plaque. BMC Oral Health. 2012;12(3):1-6.

88. Oliveira MJL, Martins CC, Paiva SM, Tenuta LMA, Cury JA. Estimated Fluoride Doses from Toothpastes Should be Based on Total Soluble Fluoride. Int. J. Environ. Res. Public Health.2013;10:5726-5736.

89. Ramazani N,Ahmadi R,Heidari Z, Hushmandi A. The Effect of Calcium Pre-Rinse on Salivary Fluoride After 900 ppm Fluoride Mouthwash: A Randomized Clinical Trial. J Dent (Tehran) . 2013;10(4):376-382.

90. Alamoudi SA,Pani SC,Alomari M. The Effect of the Addition of Tricalcium Phosphate to 5% Sodium Fluoride Varnishes on the Microhardness of Enamel of Primary Teeth. Inter J Dent.2013:1-5.

91. Ozdemir-Ozenen D, Sungurtekin E, Issever H, Sandalli N. Surface roughness of fluoride-releasing restorative materials after topical fluoride application.Eur J Paediatr Dent .2013;14(1):68-72.

92. Nalbantgil D, Oztoprak M O, Cakan D G, Bozkurt K, Arun T. Prevention of demineralization around orthodontic brackets using two different fluoride varnishes. Eur J Dent. 2013;7:41-47.

93. Reilly C, Rasmussen K, Selberg T, Stevens J, Jones RS. Biofilm Community Diversity after Exposure to 0.4% Stannous Fluoride Gels. J Appl Microbiol. 2014; 117(6): 1798–1809.

94. Chi DL. Caregivers Who Refuse Preventive Care for Their Children: The Relationship Between Immunization and Topical Fluoride Refusal. Am J Public Health. 2014;104 (7):1327-1333.

95. Aldrees AM, Albeshri SS, Alsanie IS, Alsarra IA. Assessment of fluoride concentrations in commercially available mouthrinses in central Saudi Arabia. Saudi Med J .2014;35 (10):1278-1282.

96. Komiyama K, Kimoto K, Taura K, Sakai O. National survey on school-based fluoride mouth-rinsing programme in Japan: regional spread conditions from preschool to junior high school in 2010. Intern J Dent. 2014; 64: 127–137.

97. Mazaheri R, Pishevar L, Keyhanifard N, Ghasemi E. Comparing the Effect of Topical Acidulated Phosphate Fluoride on Micro-Hardness of Two Fissure Sealants and One Flowable Composite. J Sch Dent. 2014; 32(2):103-110.

98. Alani BW, Qasim AA. The effect of topical fluoride products on surface microhardness of enamel of primary teeth. International Journal of Enhanced Research in Science Technology & Engineering. 2014;3(9):147-153.

99. Pinto SCS, Bandeca MC, Pinheiro MC, Cavassim R, Tonetto MR, Borges AH, Sampaio JE. Preventive effect of a high fluoride toothpaste and arginine-carbonate toothpaste on dentinal tubules exposure followed by acid challenge:a dentine permeability evaluation. *BMC* Res Notes.2014;7(385):1-6.

100. Sebastian ST, Siddanna S. Total and Free Fluoride Concentration in Various Brands of Toothpaste Marketed in India. J. clin. diagn. res.2015;9(10): ZC09-ZC12.

101. Itaborahy R, Machado FC, Elias GP,Ribeiro LC, Ribeiro RA. Clinical Effectiveness of Two Commercial Fluoride Varnish Formulations on the Control of White Spot Lesion in Primary Teeth: A Pilot Study. Brazilian Research in Pediatric Dentistry and Integrated Clinic.2015;15(1):41-48.

102. Bansal R, Bansal T. A Comparative Evaluation of the Amount of Fluoride Release and Re-Release after Recharging from Aesthetic Restorative Materials: An in vitro Study. J. clin. diagn. res. 2015;9(8): ZC11-ZC14.

103. Rao BSR,Moosani GKR,Shanmugaraj M, Kannapan B,Shankar BS, Ismail PMS. Fluoride Release and Uptake of Five Dental Restoratives from Mouthwashes and Dentifrices. J Int Oral Health. 2015; 7(1):1-5.

104. Bahrololoomi1 Z, Lotfian M. Effect of Diode Laser Irradiation Combined with Topical Fluoride on Enamel Microhardness of Primary Teeth. J Dent (Tehran).2015;12(2): 85 -89.

105. Suvarna GS , Nadiger RK , Shetty O. Effect of Topical Fluoride on Surface of Cast Titanium and Nickel-Chromium: An In Vitro Study. jdt.tums.ac.ir. 2015; 12(6):398-408.

106. Jessica L Milburn J L el al. Substantive Fluoride Release from a New Fluoride Varnish Containing CXP. Dentistry. 2015;5(350):2-6.

107. Valério R A et al. CO2 Laser and Topical Fluoride Therapy in the Control of Caries Lesions on Demineralized Primary Enamel. The ScientificWorld Journal.2015:1-6.

108. Hendaus M A el al.Parental preference for fluoride varnish: a new concept in a rapidly developing nation. Dovepress J.2016;10:1227–1233.

109. Byeon S M,Lee M H,Bae T S. The effect of different fluoride application methods on the remineralization of initial carious lesions.Aust Dent J.2016;41(2):121-129.

110. Jones S,Burt B A, Petersen P E,Lennon M A. The effective use of fluorides in public health. Bulletin of the World Health Organization 2005;83(9):670-676.

111. Levy S M. An Update on Fluorides and Fluorosis. J Can Dent Assoc.2003; 69(5): 286–291.

112. Grget K R,Peros K,Sutej I,Basic K. The cariostatic mechanisms of fluoride. Acta Medica Academica.2013;42(2):179-188.